Bicycling

MAXIMUM OVERLOAD FOR CYCLISTS

ALSO BY
ROY M. WALLACK

A RADICAL

STRENGTH-BASED PROGRAM

FOR IMPROVED SPEED

AND ENDURANCE

IN HALF THE TIME

Bicycling

MAXIMUM OVERLOAD FOR CYCLISTS

JACQUES DeVORE AND ROY M. WALLACK

RODALE.

RODALE *wellness*

Live happy. Be healthy. Get inspired.

Sign up today to get exclusive access to our authors, exclusive bonuses,
and the most authoritative, useful, and cutting-edge information on health, wellness,
fitness, and living your life to the fullest.

Visit us online at RodaleWellness.com
Join us at RodaleWellness.com/Join

Notice: The information in this book is meant to supplement, not replace, proper
exercise training. All forms of exercise pose some inherent risks. The editors and
publisher advise readers to take full responsibility for their safety and know their limits.
Before practicing the exercises in this book, be sure that your equipment is
well-maintained, and do not take risks beyond your level of experience, aptitude,
training, and fitness. The exercise and dietary programs in this book are not intended
as a substitute for any exercise routine or dietary regimen that may have been
prescribed by your doctor. As with all exercise and dietary programs,
you should get your doctor's approval before beginning.

Mention of specific companies, organizations, or authorities in this book
does not imply endorsement by the author or publisher, nor does mention of specific
companies, organizations, or authorities imply that they endorse this book, its author,
or the publisher. Internet addresses and telephone numbers given in this book were
accurate at the time it went to press.

Rodale books may be purchased for business or promotional use or for special sales.
For information, please write to:
Special Markets Department, Rodale Inc., 733 Third Avenue, New York, NY 10017.

Bicycling is a registered trademark of Rodale Inc.

Printed in the United States of America

Rodale Inc. makes every effort to use acid-free ∞, recycled paper ♻.

Book design by Joanna Williams

Photographs by Haldane Morris, except for page 100 by Roy M. Wallack

Library of Congress Cataloging-in-Publication Data is on file with the publisher.

ISBN-13 978–1–62336–774–9   paperback

Distributed to the trade by Macmillan

2   4   6   8   10   9   7   5   3   1   paperback

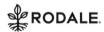 RODALE.

Follow us @RodaleBooks on

We inspire health, healing, happiness, and love in the world. Starting with you.

Jacques:

To my mother,
Madelyn DeVore,
who always told me
to seek knowledge

Roy:

To my irrepressible
dad, Norm Wallack, 88,
who's never lifted
a weight but says
he might start now

CONTENTS

INTRODUCTION

Rewriting the Rules of Endurance

<u>Maximum Overload offers all-day Maximum Sustainable Power (MSP) on reduced training time by taking cyclists to a place they never imagined they'd go: the weight room.</u>

In March 2013, in the steep Pyrenees Mountains that separate Spain and France, pro bike racer Dave "DZ" Zabriskie was ecstatic. Although not a top-10 finisher at any stage of the 7-day Volta a Catalunya (Tour of Catalonia), which included 2 days of tough summit finishes above 6,500 feet, the 34-year-old had raced far above his early-season expectations. A champion time trialist and the first American to win stages at all three of the biggest European tours (France, Italy, and Spain), DZ was never in great shape early in the season, was not a great natural climber, and was coming off a 6-month suspension for doping a decade earlier on one of Lance Armstrong's teams. But when he got on the phone, he was beyond happy.

"I kept up on the climbs!" he raved. "I wasn't gassing out on the hills. I'm sustaining my power. I'll be ready for the Tour of California [an upcoming race he'd previously finished second in four times]. The weight lifting is working."

What? *Weight lifting?*

Yes, you read that correctly. Zabriskie had been pumping iron—something competitive cyclists simply don't do, and cycling coaches have expressly warned against for a century. "Riders ride. Weights make a cyclist heavy and slow," they say, advising riders to stay away from weights at all costs (except maybe a little "core work" in the off-season). But Zabriskie, at the tail end of an impressive career with little to lose by trying something new, took a leap of faith—and something crazy happened: His power in watts on the bike jumped up—way up, a whopping 15 percent in just 4 months—while his body weight went down. Not surprisingly, his climbing was way better. On hilly training rides in the Santa Monica Mountains, he wore out Christian Vande Velde, one of his Garmin-Sharp teammates, normally a much better climber. At an age when improvement simply does not happen to the normal pro cyclist, DZ was getting better, all because he was doing two or three workouts a week of weight lifting—while riding less!

But he wasn't doing just any old three sets of 10 reps in the gym. Trying to improve his ability to sustain power longer, Zabriskie was using Maximum Overload, the world's first weight-lifting program designed specifically for cyclists.

Maximum Overload establishes a new paradigm that promises to revolutionize how people train for cycling. Using heavy weights to fire and harden the key mover muscles of cycling in short, taxing, and methodical workouts that increase the rider's ability to sustain power longer, it offers the Holy Grail of training: better performance in less workout time. And the benefits don't end there.

Specifically, Maximum Overload gives you:

- **Improved power**—so you get more out of each pedal stroke.

- **Sustained power from start to finish**—known here as Maximum Sustainable Power (MSP). By building more powerful muscle fibers, you stay fresher all day. More MSP means you are able to work less in the first half of the race and keep your speed on second-half hills and surges without gassing out in the last miles.

- **Less total workout time.** A 40-minute Maximum Overload workout can replace hours of saddle time—and improve upon it. You can cut your total training time dramatically.

- **Quick results** (often within a month or two), which keep motivation high. Grinding it out in the gym for hours is no one's idea of fun. Between massage and physical therapy, who has time? Maximum Overload gets you in and out in an hour—and in as little as 40 minutes once you're fully trained.

- **Faster recovery than typical weight workouts.** The unique combination of heavy weight and small clusters of reps is less taxing on your muscles than traditional high-intensity, high-volume programs.

- **Better form.** Fresher muscles maintain a more efficient body position and pedal stroke.

- **Fewer injuries.** The Maximum Overload protocol reduces the risks of traditional heavy weight lifting. It focuses not just on the weights, but on straightening out and protecting the whole infrastructure from overuse injuries through a step-by-step warm-up and injury-prevention movements before the big lifts.

- **An antiaging effect.** Heavy weight lifting is known to stave off the decline in muscle and bone mass associated with both aging and cycling—issues of special concern to those approaching or past age 50.

Granted, those are big, sexy promises that sound almost too good to be true—especially since they claim to apply to cyclists across the board—racer and century rider, young and old. But Los Angeles–based Jacques DeVore, Maximum Overload's inventor and the coach at the other end of Zabriskie's phone call, says they are nothing new. Other sports have been using the performance-enhancing power of weight training for years.

"Cycling is actually way behind the curve," says DeVore, a cycling coach, masters racer, strength and conditioning coach, and owner of the prestigious Sirens and Titans Fitness gym in West LA. "Basketball players, soccer players, baseball players, golfers, rowers, skiers—you name it—they all engage in vigorous weight-lifting programs today.

"Ever wonder why today's high-flying NBA players look like bodybuilders next to old videos of Magic Johnson and Larry Bird? Because they are doing serious lifting. And you can bet they wouldn't be doing it if it slowed them down. Weights are taking them to new levels," he says. "Every athlete who comes to me knows that if he was fresher in the fourth quarter, he'd win. That freshness is the result of raising what I call your Maximum Sustainable Power (MSP). And the best way to do that is with weights."

That's because, done right, weight lifting does a lot more

than make you stronger. It gives you the ultimate tools for survival in a competitive world: quickness, speed, and power (the ultimate metric because it combines strength and speed). And even though skinny endurance athletes and their clueless coaches might disagree, weight training is particularly beneficial for endurance activities, because it can help to develop the MSP necessary to fight what DeVore calls "second-half deterioration"—the typical slowdown on the last miles and last hills of the day. And, done right, weight training can help you fight it even better than riding itself.

Whether you're a century rider or stage racer, you know about second-half deterioration. On a course with six major climbs, it's the flagging attempts to get up the fifth and sixth climbs as fast as you did the first—and to keep up with surges in the pack. In a criterium race, it's the increasingly desperate efforts required to bridge to the break and keep up in the final sprint. Technically, the deterioration is due to a marked decline in sustainable power—which DeVore believes can be addressed by strengthening the muscles.

"In a long event, it's typically the muscles that give out, not the heart and lungs," he says. "It's a double whammy. With your muscles fatigued on the last hills of the day, they not only can't produce the same power they did earlier in the race but can't hold form. Your knees splay out; your pedal stroke goes from a rigid piston to a noodle. Unable to fire fully or accurately, your power drops off the table." As the hours and hill climbs and hard efforts go by, you slow down. You poop out.

DeVore emphasizes that although you may get a little faster through Maximum Overload training, raw absolute speed is NOT the main issue here.

"The key to going faster on a bike is not necessarily going ... ter, but simply not slowing down," he says. "It isn't how fast you are, but how much of that speed you can hold throughout the day.

"If your legs have what I call Maximum Sustainable Power (MSP), you will hold more of your speed than a faster guy—and in the end, you will beat him." In other words, as the speed demons of the first half slow down in the second, those with steady, fatigue-resistant power will keep on truckin'.

That's why Zabriskie was so excited. In Catalonia, early in his training cycle and unsure of his fitness, he was keeping his speed from the beginning to the end of the race.

Counterintuitively, DeVore found that the best place to build this wondrous MSP, which deeply hardens and strengthens the muscles against fatigue and deterioration, is not on the bike but in the weight room. The reason why weights are so effective is one word: OVERLOAD.

In a nutshell, weights work by concentrating an extreme stress—i.e., an overload—on your muscles that is far beyond what normal movements of life and sport can do. In a process known as supercompensation, the overload actually temporarily damages the muscles with microtears, sending alarm signals to the brain to rebuild them to be stronger, faster, and more resilient for the next go-round. The body is an amazing self-improving machine; you just need to give it the right stimulus. As you increase the overload, the muscles are stressed more and rebuilt even stronger and faster. If you can figure out a way to safely "maximize" the overload—i.e., push yourself to the limit without getting injured—you'll get the best increases in sustainable power. Hence the title and ultimate goal of this book: Maximum Overload training, which builds the Golden Ticket of endurance, MSP.

Sounds logical, right? However, all of this begs the question: If weight training has been commonly used for years in all manner of sports, even among true endurance athletes like rowers and cross-country skiers, and now is even being begrudgingly tolerated by some in the cycling world, why hasn't anyone stepped forward with a definitive plan until now? In other words, why has cycling been in the dark—and why should you listen to Jacques DeVore?

Two reasons: fear of weight gain and something DeVore calls "the Gap." First, there is legitimate fear of putting on weight, whether it be fat or muscle. Since power-to-weight ratio is everything in cycling (the gold standard for a top pro is 5-plus watts per kilogram of weight), a few extra pounds without additional power will definitely make you slower on a hill climb. Cyclists, looking at bodybuilders and CrossFitters, see big bulky muscles and assume that weight training and more muscle will make them slower. They also note that big muscles don't appear to speed them up. When do you ever see a bodybuilder hammering a bike at 27 mph?

Second, there's the Gap. "Cycling coaches usually know next to nothing about strength training, and strength coaches know little about cycling," says DeVore. "No one knows both, and therefore they don't know how to ideally tailor weights and power training to the needs of the sport."

Well, it turns out that DeVore knows both.

A former collegiate wrestler and power lifter, a credentialed National Strength and Conditioning Association

(NSCA) strength and conditioning coach, longtime masters bike racer, and elite-level cycling coach, DeVore was a successful commodities trader in the 1980s and 1990s who had a passion for cycling and strength training. He began experimenting with weight training to fight his own age-related cycling slowdown, borrowing some principles from power lifting, a weight-class sport in which competitors try to gain strength without size—which is exactly what cyclists need. Impressed by the fatigue resistance and hill-climbing prowess he appeared to gain as a result of a couple months of weight training, DeVore opened a gym and began working with cyclists, runners, and triathletes, including a national team cyclist who a decade later would go on to medal in the London Olympics. When Zabriskie came along in late 2012, DeVore had a name and a structure for his training plan and a willing world-class guinea pig to try it out on.

Maximum Overload, which maximizes the overload in a cycling-specific way that leads to improvements in MSP without adding weight, was ready for prime time.

WHAT YOU'LL FIND IN THIS BOOK

Taking Maximum Overload public, the plan in this book not only shows cyclists the benefits of weight training but also takes the randomness out of it for all athletes. It lays out a step-by-step training plan, with tutorials on all the exercises and a critical do-it-yourself assessment that allows you to coach yourself. We can't overemphasize the importance of the assessment; all people have structural issues that are exacerbated by aging and cycling itself. You cannot lift heavy weight safely with your body out of balance.

We'll save the details about the Maximum Overload program for Chapter 1, but here's a brief overview. While the full plan includes unique spins on intervals, recovery, LSD (long slow distance) training, and diet, the magic happens with the 40- to 60-minute Maximum Overload weight-lifting and power-training sessions that give the program its name. They can replace several cycling workouts per week in your off-season training (valuable for people who live in bad weather states and darkness) and even several in season, depending on your competitive level.

The keys to Maximum Overload are the *right exercises* and a *unique overload protocol that utilizes numerous sets in small batches.* That allows you to safely and comfortably lift a great quantity of heavy weight and power exercises without hating life, passing out, risking injury, spending all evening in the gym, and destroying your recovery for the next day.

The overload protocol, which we think will rewrite the rules of training for power in the gym as well as supercharge endurance athletes, can be used with any exercises and tailored to any sport. For cyclists, of course, the exercises target the mover muscles of cycling (posterior chain, quads, hamstrings, glutes, and ancillary muscles) and the supporting back and core. DeVore initially experimented with several types of deadlifts and one-legged presses, which became mainstays of the program, and settled on explosive weighted walking lunges as the ultimate transferable leg-centric power exercise. For variety and practicality, the program can work (with varying degrees of effectiveness) with alternatives such as plyo box jumps, thrusters, wall balls, and other familiar exercises, as long as they follow the Maximum Overload protocol.

At his West LA gym, DeVore works his personal clients and pro athletes with several sophisticated, rarely seen machines that allow for unique jumps and posterior chain activation. In addition to deadlifts and walking lunges, Zabriskie trained extensively on an air-resistance isokinetic machine that measured power output in standing jumps. For fun, this book shows these rare machines, but the basic Maximum Overload workout described here is a do-it-yourself version that utilizes standard equipment that you can find at your local gym or even at home.

The key point of the book is that improvements in your maximum weight lifted for certain exercises have a strong correlation to increased power performance on the bike. Zabriskie hadn't done a great deal of heavy weight training like this before he started working with DeVore, although he had decent upper-body strength and could do five-plus pull-ups—rare for a cyclist. But like all cyclists, he was lower-body–centric. A dedicated worker, he made impressive progress from December to March, raising his deadlift max from 150 pounds to 245, increasing his power on the bike by about 15 percent, and dropping the weight of his 6-foot body from 168 pounds to 154.

"It was unheard of for a guy at his age to make that kind of improvement in such a short period of time," said DeVore.

Maximum Overload worked for Zabriskie. The increased strength, power, and ability to hold maximum power in his muscles got him up the early Catalonia climbs with less effort, keeping those same muscles relatively fresher for the climbs at the end of the day—the MSP that is Maximum Overload's goal. Unfortunately, DZ's dreams went unrealized when he crashed at the Tour of California, broke his collarbone, couldn't ride the Tour de France, and retired.

Fortunately, DeVore has been busy training many more endurance athletes in his Maximum Overload program. We were thrilled to have the opportunity, as the research and writing of the book commenced, to work with the great three-time Olympian John Howard and his protégé Denise Mueller, 43, a former 15-time junior national champion whom Howard was training to set an astounding 150-plus mph land speed record on the Bonneville Salt Flats. (Howard had set a record of 152.2 mph riding in the vortex of a rocket car in 1985; under tougher conditions, Mueller almost matched that and attributed some of her success to Maximum Overload, as you'll see in Chapter 8.) You will find many observations we gleaned from Howard, Mueller, and other DeVore bike-racer clients in these pages.

Thank you for your interest in exploring this new frontier of cycling training. The efficacy of weight training to improve power for all athletes—including endurance athletes—is proven by results and science, which we will cite in the book. And as for the best type of weight and power training, we believe that Maximum Overload is a game changer that will rewrite the rules of endurance, making weight training a must-do for cyclists at all levels who want to ride stronger and longer—and don't want to be left behind.

Jacques DeVore and Roy M. Wallack
January 2017

THE MAXIMUM OVERLOAD REVOLUTION

Cyclists avoid weights like the plague. But what if weight training could raise your Maximum Sustainable Power (MSP)—and make you fatigue resistant and faster on less training time?

On May 7, 2016, the day before Mother's Day, Denise Mueller, a 43-year-old Category 2 bike racer and mother of three, won the venerable Barrio Logan Grand Prix criterium in San Diego, beating not only two dozen Cat 1s and pro riders, but women 10 to 20 years younger than her.

Jaws dropped. Eyeballs popped. This simply does not happen!

After 50 minutes and 19 laps, it came down to a sprint. "I actually just walked away from everyone!" said Mueller. "I opened a gap and didn't feel maxed out. I just pulled away. I was sort of stunned."

The second-place finisher, a pro 15 years Mueller's junior, walked up afterward and said, "Nice sprint." Mueller's coach, the great John Howard, excitedly ran up and said, "You've leveled up! Your baseline power is way up!"

What happened?

"It's the Maximum Overload!" said Mueller. "My Maximum Overload training in the gym is the real secret to my win today! Maximum Overload works."

Maximum Overload works. That's a phase you'll be hearing a lot in the coming years. From the Introduction, you saw that the Maximum Overload weight-lifting program worked for pro rider Dave Zabriskie in the Tour of Catalonia, pushing his Maximum Sustainable Power (MSP) through the roof. It's worked for dozens of cyclist and triathlete clients of Jacques DeVore, Maximum Overload's inventor. It worked for John Howard, who says it gave him more power at a lower heart rate with better control—allowing him to maintain and even slightly increase his speed in his late 60s. And it worked at the Barrio Logan crit for Mueller, a long-forgotten former 15-time national junior champion who was preparing to vault back onto the cycling world's radar screen the following September with a speed record attempt on the Bonneville Salt Flats.

Mueller, whom you'll see pictured in these pages working out with Howard in DeVore's Sirens and Titans Fitness gym in West LA, was an ideal guinea pig for Maximum Overload. Months before, highly motivated by her planned record attempt (she would ultimately reach 147.7 mph—see Chapter 8), she had listened closely as DeVore explained a concept that many in the cycling world would say was crazy.

"In most instances, it is a lack of muscular power, not a lack of aerobic training, that is the missing link to take most cyclists to the next level. And how do you get that power? Indoors—without a bike, using weights and power training."

DeVore told Howard and Mueller the hard truth: She was 43, old for a bike racer; she couldn't dramatically raise her power to levels she would need by more training on the bike; and she couldn't train any harder than she already was. But with strength and power training, she could recruit and strengthen far more of her own muscle fibers and build new ones. He said it would be analogous to "adding domestiques to your own body." Like being a team leader on a hill climb conserving her energy on a four-man break, he said, you won't blow up your muscles because you're keeping some of the fibers fresher for later.

She bought it. Mueller and Howard began working with DeVore in early 2016. A self-described gym rat who stayed in shape via running, triathlon, and gym work through two decades of bike-racing–free child raising after her success as a junior, Mueller followed DeVore's do-it-yourself program to the letter. She religiously did Maximum Overload's warm-ups, core exercises, and key mover-muscle exercises—explosive weighted walking lunges for power and deadlifts and single-leg presses for strength—in her local Encinitas gym for 45 minutes twice a week in the first 2 months (to build her strength and maximum power base), then once a week thereafter (to maintain and raise her MSP). She did not deviate from the prescribed workout sequence and rest protocol of the Maximum Overload program. And as her cumulative power overload rose in the gym, so did her sustainable power on the bike.

"Overload"—a word you will see a lot of here—has been a mainstay of sports training forever. For a muscle to strengthen and perform better, it has to be stressed with greater-than-normal resistance. The greater the overload, the stronger it is rebuilt. Muscle and aerobic systems work identically: Lift a heavy weight and your body dispatches signals and hormones that make it easier to lift the same weight next time. Sprint all out for 100 yards enough times and your body rebuilds your legs, lungs, and capillaries to cover the distance faster next time.

While overload is not a new idea, DeVore's big idea—proven in numerous university studies (see Chapter 8)—was that strength improvements built by weight lifting can give endurance athletes more sustainable power output and improved performance.

In fact, he says that a properly structured weight-training and bike-training overload can improve your ability to train aerobically at higher levels than aerobic training can by itself. In many athletes, weights improve muscular efficiency so much that they reduce the time they need to train aerobically. Spitting in the face of conventional wisdom, he says proper weight training won't slow a cyclist down or cause weight gain or injuries, as cycling coaches have thought for years. In fact, if properly designed, he says it'll do exactly the opposite.

DeVore was not surprised to see that when Mueller's cumulative overload and her ability to sustain maximum power grew in the gym, so did her performance on the bike.

A key point: This doesn't mean that Mueller's speed suddenly rose from 24 to 34 mph. It meant that she was able to hold 24 mph longer.

Mueller didn't win that day in San Diego because she was necessarily any faster than the other women in a head-to-head sprint, says DeVore. She won because, in the last mile, she still had more gas in the tank than they did—meaning she was able to hold her MSP longer. In fact, she had so much power left that it surprised her—she was undertrained on the bike due to a respiratory infection 3 weeks earlier and had eight stitches in her foot from a fall 3 days before. Nonetheless, she'd kept doing her deadlifts, one-legged presses, and explosive weighted walking lunges. By the end of the race, her muscles had power when she needed it. They were fresher than her rivals' were.

Yes, Maximum Overload will give you a nicer physique, improve your posture, revive age-shriveled muscle mass and bone density, and confer important health and longevity benefits. It's literally a lifesaver for people over 50, rebuilding wasted bones and muscles. It's a time-saver that allows riders to improve but still have a life. It will even increase your top-end power and speed a little.

But its key selling point to most riders is that it speeds you up because you don't slow down.

Why? Because your body has upgraded its muscles to produce more power longer.

In trying to figure out a way to squeeze more performance out of the same genetics, DeVore specifically designed Maximum Overload to target what he felt was the bane of all endurance athletes: "second-half deterioration," the fatigue-born slowdown in the latter part of an endurance event. It is caused by the inability of the muscles to produce higher percentages of maximum power longer.

"The more sustainable power you can give your muscles, the less hard they have to work on the first, second, third, and fourth climbs of the day," he says. "That keeps them fresher for the later climbs and hard efforts."

So after 50 hard minutes at the Barrio Logan Grand Prix, on Mueller's 19th and final climb, she simply hadn't beat up her legs as much as the other women had. She had the ability to produce a higher percentage of her maximum power at the end of the race than the other women.

That's how you win a race. It's not always the fastest sprinter who wins, but the fastest sprinter at the end of the race.

Blasted repeatedly by Maximum Overload for months in the gym, Mueller's muscles were hardened, resilient, and less fatigued than usual because she was literally working less than everyone else on the first 18 laps. The additional muscle-fiber activation that this training employs allows the muscular domestiques she'd added in the weight room to share the load, keeping her MSP intact. So while the other racers were pooped out on the last climbs, Mueller wasn't—at least not as much.

Although competing against younger pros and Category 1s with better résumés, Mueller was fresher. With the finish line approaching, her less-fatigued muscle fibers had more left to give. On the last climb, she left her competitors in the dust.

Even Howard, her coach, had to admit that there was only one reason for that: Maximum Overload. "There's no other explanation; it was the only change in her training," said the US Cycling Hall of Famer. Actually, there was one other change: She had been riding *less*.

Mueller, who at that point was Maximum Overloading just once a week as dictated by the program's MSP training phase, is a believer. Her power was up by 12 percent on Spin-Scan tests—in the same ballpark as the 15 percent gain in power experienced by Dave Zabriskie 2 years before. And she wasn't done yet.

Who would have believed that you can actually get faster and more powerful on your bike by lifting weights and power training—and riding your bike less?

As you'll see next, weight training has been surprisingly effective for athletes in all realms of sport for the last couple decades. Cycling, which has had a long-standing bias against weights, is very late to the party. But as more Maximum Overload stories like Mueller's leak out, we're betting it'll catch up fast.

The following sections discuss the evolution of weights in sports and the historical resistance of the cycling world to strength training. It also describes the research that led DeVore to come up with the unique "mini-sets plus rest" protocol of Maximum Overload, why the program is a time-saver, and why we think it'll be a requirement someday for anyone who wants to win.

For published studies of weight training's positive effect on the performance of endurance athletes and the bone and muscle protection it offers for older riders, please see Chapter 8.

ATHLETES IN MOST SPORTS TODAY LIFT WEIGHTS. CYCLISTS ARE NEXT

What if everything you know about fitness is wrong?

For years, football and baseball players lay on the field and did pregame static stretching. Then they found out that static stretching loosened the joints and reduced power output. Now people do active, "dynamic" stretching, if they stretch at all.

For decades, the US government recommended low-fat/no-fat foods and okayed sugar. Now, in opposition to current guidelines, its own scientist-staffed Dietary Guidelines Advisory Committee says sugar and refined carbs are bad and saturated fat is alright (see page 206). On top of that, nobody carbo-loads anymore for endurance events.

For generations, high jumpers cleared the bar with their bodies facing the ground. Then, in 1968, American Dick Fosbury won an Olympic gold medal by jumping over the bar facing up, with his back clearing the bar. Overnight, every high jumper learned the Fosbury Flop.

In 1989, American Greg LeMond won the Tour de France on the last day by using an aerobar, used beforehand only by triathletes and ignored by bike racers. The next year, all cyclists did their time trials with aerobars.

Sacred cows are killed in sports and life all the time. Better ideas replace old ones, sometimes overnight, sometimes glacially. Weight training is one of those better ideas, revolutionizing some sports.

Cycling, where weights have been taboo for generations, will be next.

You wouldn't know that by the current cycling landscape. Most cyclists never set foot in the weight room. Their coaches think it will make them heavy and slow. A lot of European cyclists won't even carry their own luggage for fear of putting on muscle and body weight, which they think will reduce their speed and reaction time, wreck coordination, and add too much weight. But the prevailing wisdom can change fast; 20 years ago, basketball players were skinny, baseball players were fat, soccer players were tiny waifs, and golfers had dad bods (imagine Jack Nicklaus versus Tiger Woods in the UFC Octagon). Today, muscles are everywhere in almost every sport, and weight lifting is a key part of training. In fact, the steroids scandal in baseball came about because the benefits of strength and power were so pronounced that sluggers—and some pitchers, too—couldn't get enough.

Endurance sports are virtually the last weight-training holdout. Cyclists (outside of track riders) are true weight-training virgins, clueless about what it can do for them. But many of the lessons of other sports apply to an endurance sport like cycling. One of the most important on the list is what Denise Mueller experienced that day in San Diego: Fresh legs = longer MSP.

MSP is a big part of many popular sports, even though you may not think of it right away. In basketball, the best player may not be the one who can jump the highest or shoot the best; it's the one who keeps jumping and shooting well all 48 minutes of the game with no decline in ability to execute. In boxing, the best fighter is usually the one with fresher legs who can keep punching hard and maintaining his maximum power in the 12th round. In football, it's the quarterback with the zing in his arm in the fourth quarter and the receiver who still has the spring in his legs to run a precise route at top speed and then make the leaping end zone catch. The winner is not necessarily the one with the most power, but the one who holds the highest percentage of his maximum power the longest.

That's Maximum Sustainable Power. It wins.

You could actually extend the MSP concept to months— or decades. Kobe Bryant scored 60 points in his last game in 2016, but retired at age 36 in part because his muscles weren't what they used to be; they lacked the maximum sustainable power to play back-to-back games at a high level anymore.

If there was a MSP god, it probably was Michael Jordan, a true weight-training pioneer. Frustrated by the Bulls' failure to get past the Detroit Pistons in the playoffs in the late '80s, and specifically his manhandling by the Pistons' outstanding defensive guard Joe Dumars, Jordan always felt rundown late in the year. So he decided to do weight workouts in season, not just in the off-season. His legendary, early-morning "Breakfast Club" workouts in his home's basement gym, beginning in 1990 under the direction of trainer Tim Grover, kept his power up through the playoffs. Lifting heavy every day definitely did not ruin his shot. In the '90s, Jordan won six titles in eight seasons, with the last in 1998, when he retired at age 34. He un-retired 3 years later and averaged more than 20 points a game in two seasons with the Washington Wizards at age 38 and 39.

Coincidence? Hardly. Late in the race, late in the season, late in a career, late in life, weight training to increase power pays off. It's no surprise that basketball players look so muscular nowadays—they want to be like Mike.

In cycling, it's not the absolute fastest rider or guy with the highest VO2 max (maximal oxygen-delivery capability) who wins the bike race. It's the guy who can hold the highest percentage of his sprint or MSP the longest. All things being equal, if you can hold your power better than your competitor, you will slowly make gains throughout the event. And, if need be, you'll have more left for a final burst at the end.

So, the longer the event, the more important the role of MSP. If you look at the fastest and slowest riders in the Tour de France, the difference in their speeds (both average and top speed) is relatively small. But multiply that difference over 23 days and hundreds of hours, and the gap is huge. If an Ironman triathlete can hold 2 percent more power over 8-plus hours, he or she wins—big. If a Tour de France rider can do that for 23 days . . .

For example: What if Mark Cavendish, a super sprinter but not the best time trialist, could hold a higher percentage of his sprint speed throughout the race? What if he could sustain more of his power? To be a Tour de France contender, riders have to be able to do a lot of things: Climb, time-trial, pace line, sprint, stay with and reel in competitors when they surge. This requires the ability to hold the highest percentage of their maximum power throughout the day, not just for a sprint. For Cavendish to contend for the Yellow Jersey, he needs to do something to push up his overall MSP (not just maximum power)—such as Maximum Overload. As Denise Mueller proved, it might even help him sprint better.

WHY CYCLING IS
A WEIGHT-LIFTING VIRGIN

You have to wonder: If it is well known that other sports have been using weight training for years, why is cycling so far behind the eight ball?

The first reason is power-to-weight ratio. It's a proven fact that gains in weight slow riders precipitously, especially on climbs. It lowers your power-to-weight ratio. There is a long-standing belief, probably from watching too many Arnold Schwarzenegger movies, that weight training puts on body weight.

However, it is also a fact that if a weight-training program is designed properly, weight gain doesn't have to happen. With the right weight, exercises, and rep sequence, riders will not gain weight, but can actually lose pounds while gaining strength—due to fat loss. The Maximum Overload plan, borrowing principles of powerlifting (whose athletes do not want weight gain because they compete in weight classes), uses a heavy weight/low-reps protocol that allows you to recruit more muscle fibers without putting on extra pounds. Besides the limited hypertrophy of powerlifting-style training, any muscle weight gain is replaced by concurrent fat loss, which occurred with both Zabriskie and Mueller. That's a common side effect of adding lean body mass, which is considered by many a key to general health—along with looking better naked.

The other reason for the lack of weight-training usage in cycling is the Gap, as DeVore calls it. Cycling coaches know cycling and weight-lifting coaches know weight lifting. But since cycling coaches have a limited history of lifting weights and weight coaches don't typically ride bikes, there historically has been no one who knows both and can bridge the gap. Therefore, no one has tailored an effective weight program for cyclists.

DeVore loves to tell the story of the day in 1999 that he went to the Strength and Conditioning conference at the National Sports and Conditioning Association (NSCA) annual meeting in Las Vegas. "I look on the convention floor, and everyone is bald-headed, with no neck and a goatee," he recalls. "They're all weight lifters and strength coaches! They know next to nothing about cycling or running. They have ridden a bike maybe 100 yards on the bike path from Gold's Gym to Santa Monica. And these are the guys writing strength programs for cyclists!"

They had to write the programs because cycling coaches knew virtually nothing about weights. If you go to Interbike, the massive annual bike industry trade show, and talk to bike racers, you'll see a bunch of skinny guys who've never set foot in a gym. You won't see a booth with a pull-up bar or a squat rack or anything that relates to strength training. Most cycling coaches were bike racers—and may have never lifted a weight or written a strength program.

Bottom line: The cyclist is left in the middle. "This is the Gap—a no man's land for the endurance athlete trying to find out what to do with weights," says DeVore.

Ultimately, with few cycling strength coaches and little information about it available, the myth that strength training does not work for cyclists is perpetuated.

Yes, strength training has entered the conversation these

days. Cyclists aren't blind—they see soccer players and skiers (including endurance fiends like cross-country skiers) lifting weights like their lives depend on it. Some are doing CrossFit. But the vast majority of cyclists and their coaches wouldn't have a clue what to do with a barbell.

DeVore, however, did have a clue. In 1980, as a collegiate wrestler at UC Davis who lived in the weight room, he often ran into future six-time Hawaii Ironman triathlon winner Dave Scott, a coach of the local masters swim team. If Scott's dominance of the Ironman in the 1980s against a bunch of muscle-tone–challenged swimmers and runners was not a wake-up call for triathletes that weight training helped endurance (it wasn't—even today triathletes rarely touch weights), it was for DeVore. As he built a successful money management firm in the following decades, he remembered his conversations with Scott. While DeVore sold his practice, opened a futures trading company, toyed with powerlifting, got heavily into bike racing, and moonlighted in the fitness industry (his true love), Scott come out of retirement to finish second and fifth at the Hawaii Ironman at ages 38 and 40. It was a stunning achievement; in that era, the mid-1990s, 40 was considered ancient.

In interviews with reporters covering the triathon, like this book's cowriter, who was then an editor of *Triathlete* magazine, Scott always attributed much of his success to the power and resiliency he gained from weight training. It certainly made him a rarity in the sport—and apparently didn't mess with his power-to-weight ratio too much. As DeVore entered his 40s, he took note.

Around the time that he went to the NSCA conference,

DeVore spent time at the US Olympic Training Center—in Chula Vista, California, to get his expert cycling coaching certification. It consisted of 2 days of classes and an exam.

When the subject of weight training came up, the exercise physiologist leading one of the courses shrugged it off. "Eh—nothing shows that weight lifting enhances cycling," he said. "Strength does not increase endurance. Just do big-chainring work."

DeVore, confused, raised his hand. "If strength is not a limiting factor in endurance, then why do big-chainring work at all?"

The answer shocked him: "Uhhh, uhh, uhh—well, it's tradition," stammered the lecturer.

"He had no reasonable answer to the question 'Why?'" says DeVore. "Well, why not? Why were we not looking at this? Why don't cyclists lift weights?" There simply wasn't much research about it.

"Skiers are in the weight room like maniacs," he says. "Why are endurance athletes not undergoing this same evolution? The naysayers who tell endurance athletes not to lift have closed their minds. They hide behind tradition and have lost the curiosity to ask why."

A couple years before, DeVore had taken a strength coach exam and started managing Vert Sports Performance in Santa Monica, a high-tech gym that had supplied Keiser-made isokinetic equipment to Michael Jordan's trainer, Tim Grover.

After trying it out, Shaquille O'Neill requested that the Lakers buy the same $20,000 isokinetic air-resistance "jumping machine," in which you crouch under a padded crossbar, press it against your shoulders, and explode up against resistance. (The machines were so expensive that they didn't catch on; only rehab centers could afford them.) The machine offers resistance only on the way up. As you jump and land, it measures vertical leaping power in foot-pounds. The isokinetic machine provided a tremendous workout and was seen as a secret weapon to keep Shaq and his team fresh in the fourth quarter. The Lakers don't owe three consecutive NBA titles to their jumping machine, but it didn't hurt.

As DeVore, then in his early 40s and heavily into bike racing, began noticing an age-related decline in his speed and power numbers, he began toying with the isokinetic machine himself. Soon he was using it to train a bike-racer friend, who a decade later would go on to win a silver medal at the London Olympics. "It improved her cycling dramatically," he said.

Over time, DeVore trained many athletes on the isokinetic machine: Trinidad's four-time Olympic champion sprinter Ato Bolden, now a USA track TV commentator; NBA player Shawn Kemp; Oakland Raiders defensive tackle Regan Upshaw; New York Giants linebacker Dhani Jones; and several NFL draftees getting ready for the NFL scouting combine. A decade later, he would use it to train Dave Zabriskie.

While running Vert, DeVore started reading the translated texts of great Russian strength-training coaches—the USSR dominated powerlifting at that time and had very advanced research, which he shared at some speeches he gave on weight lifting for cyclists. (As we now know, the Eastern bloc was using more than just the weight room to enhance performance. However, many of the techniques for training design and tactics and understanding of physiology that we are just starting to use today were being used by Communist strength coaches in the late 1960s and 1970s.)

"My knowledge was rudimentary; over time it evolved," he says. "But lifting weights was helping me and others ride a bike faster. This was part of the genesis of my figuring this out. I was onto something."

Before we get into how DeVore came up with the unique Maximum Overload protocol and exercises, let's examine the broader overall question: How does a cyclist benefit from lifting weights?

WHAT WEIGHTS DO FOR CYCLISTS

Let's be honest: Lifting weights isn't as much fun as riding a bike. When you're hoisting barbells and dumbbells in the gym, there's no cool sightseeing, no endorphin high. It's nothing but hard work—grunt it out, push it hard, grind your teeth. Lifting weights is about as much fun as flossing.

But like flossing, your 5-year colonoscopy when over 50, and your IRA, weights are necessary for the short run and the long run. Weights allow you to hold power and form, the two keys to performance (discussed in more detail below). Weights can cause significant changes in your body: improvements in strength and power, biomechanical integrity, and aerobic performance, plus more resistance to injuries due to strengthening of bones and connective tissue. They let you ride less, which reduces the chance of burnout, boredom, and car accidents. They assure uninterrupted training by strengthening the muscles around the joints, which cushions them and maintains alignment. They stop the catabolic effect of aerobic monotraining, slow and reverse the muscle-mass deterioration that starts in everybody about age 35 and accelerates every decade, and can reverse the alarming bone thinning that is endemic to the sport of cycling, no matter your age. Bottom line: Weight training will keep you riding years longer, even decades longer, and increase your general quality of life.

If the long-term benefits of weight training seem too hazy, and you need a more urgent reason to start pushing iron, consider this: Strength training works quickly. One or two days a week in the weight room for a month or two—replacing 20 to 30 percent of your training time—will make you faster. Noticeably faster.

That's because improved muscle performance equals speed. More lean muscle means more force production, increased power, more energy, and better processing of oxygen and calories. Weights can make you better on the bike much faster than you can do it on the bike itself. That's because they can give you a concentrated overload that rapidly improves performance in muscle fibers.

There's the magic word again: *overload*. The more overload, the better. Overload refers to any higher-than-normal stress on your muscles and bones. If you are used to walking on flat ground, hiking up a steep hill with a 40-pound backpack would be considered an overload. If you are used to riding on flat ground, riding up a hill in the big chainring will be an overload. If you are a serious bike rider, doing heavy deadlifts will be an overload. In each case, you are subjecting your muscles to more stress than they are used to. Your body will respond by making the whole musculoskeletal system—your muscles, connective tissue, and bones—stronger.

This self-improvement process, technically known as "supercompensation," results in the overloaded body parts being rebuilt with a higher performance capacity than they had prior to the overloading. Overload can be light to heavy, or abrupt or gradual; any overload alarms your body and sets repair messages in motion. If the overload is too easy, of course, not much will happen. Maximum Overload, as you can guess, uses heavy weights to create maximum stress—and maximum gains without adding body weight. (To figure out your Maximum Overloads see "Maximum Overload Math and Exercise Correlation" on page 42).

The most timeworn but illustrative example of a gradual overload is the fabled Roman calf raise, in which a Roman gladiator's strength incrementally grows over time as he trains by lifting a calf day after day as a child until he is lifting a bull as an adult. The bottom line: Overload the body, and it comes back better.

The following is a quick rundown of the benefits of weight training for cyclists (*Note:* see Chapter 8 for some academic studies on the benefit of weight training for endurance):

1. **The ability to hold power and hold form.** Weights upgrade these two key muscle functions, delaying the second-half fatigue that slows you down and makes you slip into a sloppy, inefficient body position. Holding power refers to maintaining a consistent level of propulsion from the beginning to the end of the event, such as being able to climb the last hill of a bike race as

fast as you did the first without getting fried. Holding form refers to maintaining a consistent, sport-specific posture from the beginning to the end of the ride. That includes keeping a linear, pistonlike pedal stroke with no wasted motion and a flat, unrounded back, which keeps breathing easy and your back safe.

2. **Weights provide a huge bang for the buck,** overloading you two times at once. Besides blasting you with the sheer heaviness of the weight itself, weights supercharge the overload with an eccentric as well as a concentric contraction. Cycling is concentric, in which your quads and glutes shorten as they push the pedal. But weights force you to also work eccentrically, as the muscle lengthens with resistance as you lower the weight. That eccentric load is actually harder on your muscles, causing more microtears, which then get rebuilt stronger and subsequently improve the concentric movement as well. Although there is no eccentric load in cycling (the hamstring and momentum bring the pedal around), it turns out that the eccentric load magnifies the stress on the quads and glutes and gives them more concentric power. So an eccentric contraction helps strengthen a concentric contraction. That's one reason why riding cannot work your muscles as hard as weights can.

3. **Enhanced training on the road.** Weight training builds you up so that you can do higher overloads on the bike itself and therefore get more out of each training ride. So even on a leisurely recovery spin, you are

unwittingly putting out more power and getting an improved training effect.

4. **Better bones.** Bone health is a crucial issue for cyclists, as cycling's lack of weight-bearing impact does not cue bone growth. Combined with the sport's high loss of calcium through sweat and breathing, all cyclists are candidates for osteoporosis. The stress of weight training blasts and stresses bones as cycling does not, encouraging them to drink in more calcium to get stronger. At the very least, all cyclists should be lifting weights to protect their bones—and tendons and ligaments, too, which attach to muscles and bones and move with them. See Chapter 8 for an extensive report on the alarming bone loss suffered by cyclists who spend long hours in the saddle.

5. **Better muscle mass.** Muscles naturally shrivel with age after 35—unless you lift weights. Riding (unless you're a track rider) won't keep them robust as you age.

6. **Strength and power without more size.** Cyclists, as power-to-weight athletes, don't want more weight— and won't get it if they lift weights the Maximum Overload way. Keep in mind that there are two ways to gain strength: hypertrophy (bigger muscles) or getting more muscle fibers within each muscle to fire in a shorter period of time. To recruit those previously inactive or underused fibers (your "domestiques"), Maximum Overload borrows the methodology of powerlifters: Go heavy with low reps. Heavy weights with a low rep count causes deep muscular firing of

previously unworked fibers and avoids putting on size (hypertrophy).

- Hypertrophy is caused by doing a high rep count with moderate weights—a formula that causes a high-intensity, moderate-weight Olympic-lift workout, like CrossFit, to make both male and female athletes huge. CrossFit Games participants often look like "bodybuilders who can run fast," DeVore says, "although they're not fast enough to be really fast."
- More weight comes off, even on skinny people, as Maximum Overload sheds fat, increases your metabolism, and adds lean muscle. Weights zap fat and replace it with lighter-weight muscle, even on skinny people. As mentioned, Dave Zabriskie and Denise Mueller both lost weight while doing their Maximum Overload weight-lifting programs.

7. **Weights can fix imbalances.** You can't fix your biomechanical problems while on the bike; you just magnify them. But in the weight room, you can clearly identify and work to reduce kyphosis (slumped-forward back, shoulders, and neck) and side-to-side inequalities in strength and flexibility. Hip, shoulder, knee, and ankle mobility problems can be fixed through weight training and mobility work in the gym. That will translate into more power on the bike, greater over-loads in your Maximum Overload program, and something we all like: better looks and posture.

8. **Tremendous time-saver.** If you're not a pro athlete and have a regular family life with no time for a mas-

sage and 15 hours of riding time a week, weights are a godsend. Some of DeVore's clients (see the sidebars on pages 95, 146, and 180) claim one weight session can take the place of 2 or 3 riding days both in-season and off-season. It's ideal for those crunched for time or in the short days of winter. Zabriskie reduced his training time on the bike by 20 percent while training with DeVore.

9. **Hormonal benefits.** Heavy weight training temporarily raises your human growth hormone (HGH) and testosterone levels to support muscle growth and recovery.

10. **Anyone can do it by themselves.** Once you learn proper form and master the movement, you don't need a trainer. Weight training with the Maximum Overload system is simple and easy to follow with basic weight equipment by everyone—average folks and masters athletes, clerks at Walmart, and partners at Deloitte. Whether you are looking for higher cycling performance and/or general health, weight training works.

The bottom line? Overload is good for you. The more of it, the more you improve everything—your bones, your looks, your health at any age, and your ability to sustain maximum power on the bike. (Again, see Chapter 8 for more details on weight training's broad-based benefits for athletes.)

As DeVore slowed down on the bike in his 40s, he naturally wondered: How can I get the biggest, longest, heaviest possible overload to improve my ability to sustain my power? His

quest led to the discovery that created the Maximum Overload program and is the reason you are holding this book.

He calls it "the rest between the reps."

THE MAXIMUM OVERLOAD EPIPHANY: MINI-SETS AND REST BETWEEN THE REPS

When training for absolute power output, the convention
had always been to do three sets of 6 to 8 explosive movements with weights or body-weight exercises. Then, when
training for power endurance, the convention has been to do
as many of these explosive movements in a row as possible.

But is this the best way?

In the year 2000, DeVore didn't question the three-sets-
of-6-to-8 orthodoxy. As he started to perform his power
workouts on the aforementioned isokinetic jumping machine,
he set the velocity to a level that was his maximum power
output—100 foot-pounds—and did a set of 6 reps. That gave
him a neat total overload of 600 foot-pounds for the first set.
He did three sets of those and, utterly destroyed by the third
set, eked out a total overload of 1,800 foot-pounds of total
power. Sometimes, just to make it through the workout, he'd
have to lower the velocity to 80 foot-pounds on the third set
and end up with 1,680 foot-pounds.

Then he heard about a new product called AVAcor—and
had a lightbulb moment that caused him to reject the old
three-sets-of-6-to-8 orthodoxy and create the unique Maximum Overload training structure.

Reading a sports-performance journal, DeVore came

across an article about a radical new training aid that would be described later in the media as a "magic cooling glove" that could be "better than steroids." Actually, AVAcor was a cumbersome prototype at the time, a creation of Stanford University biology professors Dennis Grahn and Craig Heller, who theorized that cooling the palms of people who were working out would increase their performance and get them bigger overloads in each workout.

Their breakthrough discovery: Heat fatigues muscles. Keep them cool, and you perform better.

The airtight mitt used suction to circulate water over the palm in a vacuum, accelerating the palm's blood-cooling/ heat-dissipation function. The body's nonhairy skin sites— palms, soles, and face—have special blood vessels that can receive a large volume of blood and act as radiators, sending cooled blood back to the body's core and muscles. Their studies claimed that wearing AVAcor (today called Core-Control) allowed people to do 144 percent more pull-ups on a warm 95-degree day. (On a cooler 72-degree day, it didn't have as much effect.) It was said to be used by the Stanford University football team, the San Francisco 49ers, Manchester United, and the German national team during the 2014 FIFA World Cup in Brazil.

The cooling glove never set the world on fire. But the concept of cooling off the palms to quickly dissipate core muscle heat and rejuvenate the body was not junk science. It turns out that this was the first research to look at the very real effect of muscle core temperature on performance.

It resonated with DeVore, who wanted to figure out a way to get more overloads in his own isokinetic power workouts.

The lesson here was that as core muscle temperature rises, power falls. So to raise the overload, he had to stop the muscles from going into an overheated state during the workout.

His mind raced. "Why wait to get to the point where you need to cool the muscle off? Why not use preventive medicine?" he wondered. "To prevent the muscles from heating up in the first place, why not dip them in water? Heck, why not just take a quick break to let the body cool?"

And finally . . . "How about just playing with the rest between the reps?"

So there it was, DeVore's epiphany: To be able to produce maximum power longer, lower the reps, and split up each set into a series of mini-sets. After a few reps, you'd simply take a brief rest to shake out the hands and prevent the muscles from getting too hot. Theoretically, that would let you do more cumulative reps with the same heavy (or heavier) weight—giving you greater overloads longer. That should grow your Maximum Sustainable Power (MSP) much faster than the old three-sets-of-6-to-8 pattern of power training (which has suboptimal outputs as well as a smaller total overload).

He tried it. Now, instead of struggling to complete three sets of 6 straight maximal-power jumps with 100 foot-pounds of power on the isokinetic machine, he did 3 high-quality maximal-output jumps at 100 foot-pounds every 10 seconds, which built in an 8-second rest. Over 1 minute, he did six 3-jump mini-sets. Then he did two more sets just like it. And he was stunned. He was able to maintain the 100 foot-pound output for a total of 54 jumps.

"Before, I did a total of 2,800 foot-pounds in total overload. Now, I did 100 foot-pounds x 18 jumps per minute x 3 sets = 5,400 foot-pounds of total overload! This was almost twice the overload of my previous workouts! On my first try, I did 192 percent more overload at what I call my Absolute Power Output!" (APO, this programs' other major abbreviation, is your top baseline power.)

He kept experimenting: "Can I do three jumps every 10 seconds and sustain that power for longer than a minute?" His goal was to see how many total jumps he could get for the longest time at this APO—not at submaximum power.

Rest between the reps. It was that simple: no more than six or more consecutive efforts at submaximal power output. By breaking the sets into mini-sets and having the discipline to rest between the reps, you can safely raise the quantity and maintain APO. That skyrockets your overload and your MSP. With the mini-sets, you radically accelerate your body's ability to produce APO for a longer period of time. Forget a year or 6 months of weight training. With Maximum Overload workouts, you could be seeing major improvement in a month.

Ultimately, over the next couple months of resting between the reps and breaking his sets into mini-sets, DeVore got up to 4 and 5 reps per 10 seconds and reached an astounding 21,000 foot-pounds of overload during one workout on the isokinetic machine. That compares to the 2,800 foot-pounds he started with—more than seven times as much!

"Holy crap—this is unbelievable!" he told people.

He got them real excited when he also told them the single thing that they really wanted to know: "It translated to the bike. On the bike, my legs didn't tire out!"

Okay, now we're talking!

By forcing his body to spend more time at APO—its all-out 6-rep effort level—DeVore was training to delay fatigue. The body subsequently adapted by recruiting more and more soldiers (muscle fibers) for the fight. Does that mean Maximum Overload makes you "fatigue-proof"?

"That makes it sound like a hokey infomercial slogan," he grouses. "Nothing is fatigue-proof; we're human." But fatigue resistant? "Yes, I'll go for that," he says.

"Technically, it allows you to produce higher amounts of power longer before you fatigue"—meaning you can push your inevitable fatigue limit out much farther than before, ideally past the finish line.

Besides the new fatigue-resistant power in the legs, DeVore speculates that Maximum Overload causes some rise in VO_2 max, too. "I think that there is symmetry between the two, that as your body makes an adaptation to the overload, it also figures out a way to deliver more oxygen," he says. "When you're under the gun longer, the body adapts. The old way doesn't keep you under stress long enough to adapt." For the same reasons, DeVore speculates that there is a symmetry in your body between power in the gym and power in your lungs, although he has no proof of this.

While the researchers sort that out, let's get back to "the rest between the reps." It's the phrase that pays for Maximum Overload, the reason why the workout develops your MSP. With rest between the reps and mini-sets, DeVore found that he suddenly could produce huge quantities of APO for longer periods of time, eliciting a huge super-compensating response.

MINI-SET MAGIC

Once you've established your baseline APO, breaking three sets into mini-sets with rest in between each of them is the key to the Maximum Overload program's development of Maximum Sustainable Power (MSP). Here's why it works:

1. **It focuses on power.** Since Power = Strength x Speed (technically, the physics is Power = Force x Velocity), maintaining a fast speed is paramount. The mini-sets are small enough that you can keep up the velocity on each rep—unlike longer sets that cause you to slow down by the 8th or 10th rep. Your goal is to HOLD POWER—move the greatest amount of weight at the greatest amount of speed without slowing down. If you're jumping, your goal isn't to jump higher, but to maintain nearly your highest jump for more jumps. If you're doing the walking lunge, increase the steps at the same fast pace.

2. **It keeps you producing APO** (i.e., lifting heavy weights at a fast pace), not slipping down to submaximal power efforts. There are no gains from going too light and/or too slow. "Go max or go home."

3. **It leaves you fresher**—not wasted—for the next day. If you skip the rest and go to full failure, you will be wasted.

4. **It replicates the stresses of a bike race**—surviving repeated hills, surges, and hard efforts without going to failure until the final sprint. It trains your muscles to go hard all day long.

5. **The repeated short-duration explosive efforts** in the gym will limit the second-half degradation of form and power that dog everyone from racers to century riders.

6. **It reduces injury risk.**

   When do you stop? Eventually you reach a natural limit. If you can improve your ability to sustain power by 10 percent, your speed increases quickly. In 4 to 8 weeks, DeVore reports a 5 to 15 percent improvement in his clients.

In truth, resting between the reps is so simple that it seems too simple. But just go back to your old three sets of 8 or three sets of 10 and compare. It works. Maximum Overload will get you way more overload every time.

And that's what wins the race.

THE ZABRISKIE EXAMPLE

Dave "DZ" Zabriskie's power naturally dwarfed that of the average rider, but by the end of the isokinetic training with DeVore in 2013, he seemed almost supernatural. He was doing 6 jumps every 15 seconds (24 jumps per minute) and holding that pace for 4 minutes straight—a total of 96 jumps at a APO of 115 foot-pounds. That's huge—a total of 11,040 foot-pounds of overload maintaining his max power output on all the jumps. "And we did two or three sets of that," says DeVore, still marveling.

If Zabriskie's power dropped more than 10 percent on any one jump, DeVore would stop him immediately, because he didn't want DZ to put out any submaximal efforts. At that point, Zabriskie was getting too fatigued to maintain APO, at which point the body won't make the adaptation that will recruit more muscle fibers—so there is no need to continue. The body says, "No need to recruit more; we've got enough muscle fibers for a submaximal effort." That's why you must do your efforts at close to maximal effort; otherwise, the body doesn't need to make an adaptation.

"Why would you add more domestiques if no one is going up the hill fast?" says DeVore. "Your body is always trying to do the least amount of work that it can get by with—

conservation of effort. If you go submaximinal for too long in training, you'll go submaximal in a race."

Remember, what wins a bike race isn't the person with the highest VO$_2$ max, but the person sustaining the highest percentage of it the longest.

The benefits of building more resilient muscles from weight and power training will be particularly beneficial to master athletes, who maintain aerobic fitness but see APO decline. VO$_2$ max declines along with the relentless deterioration of aging. "What do they say about boxers?" says DeVore. "They lose their legs. Well, it's the same thing for cyclists. Training for improving MSP will reduce the speed at which you lose your legs."

THE DIFFERENCE BETWEEN STRENGTH AND POWER: THE KEY TO MAXIMUM OVERLOAD

Strength and power are not the same. Maximum Overload training works because it evolves from building strength to building power to building MSP.

Nothing gets DeVore more riled up than people who confuse strength and power. "They are not the same!" he will inform you in no uncertain terms.

That's because, to truly understand why Maximum Overload is so effective and why certain exercises are emphasized in certain training phases, you must understand the difference between strength and power. After all, why do we use a deadlift to warm up for an explosive weighted walking lunge—and not the other way around?

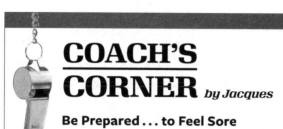

COACH'S
CORNER _by Jacques_

Be Prepared ... to Feel Sore

The phone rang. "I feel sluggish, slow, and heavy. My legs feel crappy, no snap, no bounce—I feel ehhhh," said Denise Mueller. So I told her to stay away from the Swami's Ride, the famous and furious Wednesday-evening ride in Encinitas, California, that draws rabid triathletes and bike racers like moths to flame. It wasn't as if I hadn't warned her. She was only a couple weeks into Maximum Overload training, blasting muscles she didn't even know existed before. Well, of course she was sore. Sore legs are a bitch. What do you expect?

Give it a few more weeks, I told her.

It is important that you set the proper expectations with any new training, but particularly with training that is so different from what you've been doing for years. Denise was experienced in the weight room, yet she was still sore. If you are new to weight training and power training, expect to be sore for a month—and try to savor it, because you will forget about it soon enough. Soreness is a sign that you are giving it your all in the gym—voluntarily undergoing a complete overhaul that will upgrade underutilized muscles that have been ignored for too long.

Weight training and cardio can seem like oil and water. The mix is known as "concurrent" training, and there is a legitimate physiological argument that the two impact one another negatively. Hormonally, there is actually a conflict between two hormones.

1. AMPK, released in endurance activities like long intervals and long slow distance (LSD), raises your ability to use sugar and fat for fuel and over time ups capillary density and mitochondria.
2. MTorc1, which aids protein synthesis; as this hormone increases, muscles get bigger and stronger.

And why is the walking lunge used for the Maximum Overload test and the deadlift isn't, even though the deadlift is

As it turns out, one enzyme turns off the other. But it's not a deal breaker, as some of the studies referenced in Chapter 8, which show cyclists riding faster with weight training, confirm. And you can reduce the impact of these seemingly conflicting enzymes through diet timing. The biggies:

1. Reduce your carbs the night before you do intervals, which will lower the impact of AMPK on the Maximum Overload workout to follow.

2. Eat carbs after the endurance workout if you plan to do Maximum Overload the next day. You can follow the workout with a protein drink.

But no matter what you do, expect to hurt, walk funny, start slow, and feel lethargic on the bike. My coauthor, Roy, felt this when he did the program in 2013, then called one day and told me that he finished in the top 25 percent of the 8-mile time trial up the steep Piuma Road hill climb at the recent Beverly Hills Gran Fondo—and he's usually in the bottom third. Now he laughs when friends who he's training go through it, and he tells them what I told him: The discomfort will typically pass after 3 to 4 weeks of consistent training, and you will begin to see real gains in power on the bike, with gradual increases in effectiveness and efficiency and diminished ancillary fatigue in the lower back and shoulders.

Three weeks after Denise called me, she called again, really excited. She did the Swami's Ride the night before. It was 5 weeks into her Maximum Overload training. "I could move up when I wanted, I felt more snappy—and people were commenting on it. People asked me what I was doing. They couldn't believe I was lifting weights."

a mainstay exercise of the overall Maximum Overload program?

For that matter, why does a strength exercise like a heavy deadlift or a bench press make you utter a long "uuuuughhhhh!" while a power exercise like a walking lunge or a thruster will make you blurt a short "huht!"?

Because, like DeVore said, strength and power are not the same thing.

Confused? It's understandable. The deadlift is a strength exercise whose objective is to produce the highest amount of force. Strength exercises move slowly—you grunt and groan while you agonizingly pull or push the monstrously heavy barbell or dumbbells. By contrast, the explosive weighted walking lunge is a power exercise whose objective is to move the greatest amount of weight at the highest possible speed. Using medium-weight dumbbells, you move fast—ideally exploding so fast with so much momentum as you move from step to step that sometimes your feet automatically keep going. In power exercises that thrust the bar overhead, the movement is so fast that your feet almost leave the ground and the bar keeps rising after you've stopped. The early-phase strength training builds the foundation for APO and the MSP workouts.

So strength and power exercises operate differently. Strength is the raw ability to produce force—to lift something, to press something. But power combines strength with velocity—how fast you can lift/hit something, press something. An NFL defensive lineman can grunt and groan his way to a 500-pound bench press; that's strength. But when he blasts off the line and knocks a giant offensive lineman flat on his ass, that's power. He could only do that by combining strength with velocity. As strong as the defensive lineman is, he couldn't have rung that guy's bell without lots of speed behind his strength. Pow! As in power.

"What makes you go is power," says DeVore. "We want power. Power is what wins races and scores victories in every single sport. Strength is very important, but it is a component of power. The other half of power is speed. Power ties strength and velocity into movement."

In fact, there is a simple formula for power, probably familiar to anyone who didn't sleep through the first day of physics class:

Strength x Speed = Power

Why is this formula important to know? Well, our goal with Maximum Overload is to achieve MSP in the gym and on the bike. And it gives you two factors to play with: strength and speed. The challenge here is, through trial and error, figuring out the optimal combination of strength and velocity we need to ride as fast as possible in a race or get the greatest overload during a workout in the gym. Maximum Overload helps you find out your own personal sweet spot, your optimal combination—where you produce the greatest amount of APO.

Actually, this is nothing new for you on the bike. Unknowingly, you make power decisions every few seconds, hunting for the sweet spot while on your group ride with your friends or even while riding alone. When you search for the right gear to keep up on a hill and feather between different gears while on the flats, you are trying to figure out the best combo of gears and cadence—strength and speed. You're trying to push the biggest possible gear ("strength") at the highest possible rpm ("velocity") in order to produce the MSP and speed, but there are practical limitations. If you push too big a gear, you can't spin it very fast—and your power will drop. Similarly, push too small a gear and you'll spin too much; again, your power drops. Eventually, you'll find a combination of gears and rpms that'll get you up the hill as fast as possible. And after you find your optimal gear, your sweet spot, you can hear the people behind you shifting gears in a frantic attempt to find their optimal gear to keep up with you.

Although people recoil at the sight of the words "Lance Armstrong" nowadays, DeVore believes his battles with Jan Ulrich make an instructive point. The strong Ulrich mashed a big gear with a low or approximately 80 rpm for his MSP. Armstrong, not as strong, kept up with a higher cadence of 110 rpm in a hill climb. If he went with too big of a gear too early, he'd run out of gas; unable to continue to hold the power output, he'd get dropped. This trade-off between strength and speed plays out in the weight room as weight and speed. To produce the APO the longest, you always ask the question: What weight with what velocity?

So what's the right gear in the gym for you?

Where Maximum Overload ultimately does its job is getting you that one extra gear. You know how you always say, "Crap—I wish I was strong enough or fit enough to drop one more gear"? By increasing your power in the gym and on the bike, Maximum Overload training raises your power-to-weight ratio and gets you that extra gear. It gets you more power to push the pedals harder without feeling like it's more effort than before. It lets you climb that hill one gear higher.

If you could do that, where would it put you at the end of the ride?

In the gym, we have a wide array of exercises to choose from to build both strength and power (power development can't be strictly isolated with weights; speed and strength occur together). So we narrow it down to cycling-compatible exercises that fire the same quad/hip/glute/lower-back kinetic chain of muscles that are used to push the pedals.

The deadlift leads the pack of force-producing, grunt-inducing strength exercises. A deadlift simply involves picking up a heavy weight from the floor; starting from a squatted position, you hold the bar and stand up, with the bar ending up at waist level. Arms play no role in the movement, other than holding the bar. The deadlift is superb for building cycling-compatible lower-body strength and core stability, because you can safely use very heavy weight and get a monster overload. Get in trouble? Just drop the bar or dumbbells. Remember that since the deadlift starts from a fixed, non-moving position, it's a pure strength exercise. The deadlift alone will benefit you as a cyclist, but will have minor impact on sustained speed development compared to an explosive weighted walking lunge.

On the other hand, the walking lunge, the go-to Maximum Overload test exercise for power, is ideal for developing sustainable power because it works both strength and speed in a very cycling-specific manner. In an explosive weighted walking lunge, you hold a dumbbell in each hand, step forward into a deep lunge, and rapidly "explode" forward into the next step as you move down the hallway. DeVore believes it is the best do-it-yourself power exercise available, almost as good as some specialized equipment he's used over the years, like the aforementioned isokinetic jumping machine and his current gym's rarely seen VersaPulley, sort of a rowing-machine-from-hell for your hips and quads. While the explosive weighted walking lunge clearly moves your legs slower than, say, sprints (which are also part of the comprehensive Maximum Overload plan—see Chapter 6), there's a known correlation between speed and power activities. For example, 100-meter sprinters (runners) are almost always good vertical jumpers and are helped by doing them in training. A variety of jumps are very good power activities for cyclists, although limited because they can't be easily weighted and have an injury risk factor (when you get fatigued).

For the Maximum Overload test, DeVore believes the explosive weighted walking lunge stands out among the available do-it-yourself power exercises you'll see described in Chapter 2—jumps, thrusters, push presses, power cleans, and others—because, like cycling, it is dynamic and alternate-legged and uses momentum and continuous movement. In addition, it is quite safe (just drop the dumbbells if tired), is easy to do timed and to gauge your speed, and can even be done with household items like bricks and buckets.

However, the walking lunge is a power exercise and can't hold a candle to the deadlift in terms of pure strength development. That's why the two of them work so well together in the program. The strength exercises build a foundation for the power exercises.

You see, the deadlift is a great tool for cyclists because it makes the explosive weighted walking lunge better. It gives you raw strength that'll help push pedals harder, is a super muscle-activation warm-up that grooves neuromuscular pathways for the lunge, and is good for your general health.

Bottom line: The deadlift supercharges your lunges. And the lunges supercharge your cycling.

See the connection? Strength exercises build the foundation for your power exercises—which help your cycling.

That's why the deadlift and the explosive weighted walking lunge are essential to the Maximum Overload program. They help you optimize both strength and speed/power, which together create what you need to increase your MSP.

The strength-versus-power issue affects how the Maximum Overload program plays out through the year. Because power must be developed on a foundation of strength, the off-season emphasizes strength in twice-a-week workouts. When strength begins to plateau, the strength phase transitions to the power phase, which increases the emphasis on the lunges and power exercises. As racing season develops, you reduce the strength work to maintenance and enter the once-a-week MSP phase, which has shorter workouts.

Denise Mueller followed this scenario over a 4-month period with impressive results. Her deadlift numbers rose from 170 pounds to 235 pounds—a 35 percent improvement, which actually is fairly normal for someone not experienced with weight training. (The inexperienced Zabriskie had extraordinary gains, rising from 150 to 275 pounds.) Mueller's explosive weighted walking lunge Maximum Overload workouts progressed from 15-pounds/2-minute sets to

MAXIMUM OVERLOAD
WORKOUT SUMMARY

Overview: After you've built a base of strength, you move on to the goal of Maximum Overload: building Maximum Sustainable Power (MSP). After a series of warm-up drills and preparatory core, back, and leg exercises, you begin the culmination of the workout with a Baseline APO Test, which identifies the heaviest weight with which you can do 12 steps of well-paced explosive weighted walking lunges. You then use that weight for the grand finale of Maximum Overload training, the MSP workout.

Over time, you continually retake the Baseline APO Test to raise the weight and push the MSP workout to longer durations and overloads.

1. **Baseline Power Test.** Using the heaviest possible weight that allows you to maintain enough fluid speed and momentum in which you don't get bogged down at the bottom of the step, do 12 steps (6 left-right reps) of explosive walking lunges to "failure" (the point at which you can't complete the 7th rep at full speed and control; that is, you are bogged down and stuck at the bottom of the step). Speed must be maintained on every rep, so you come off the floor fast and don't slow down and grind over the top. Use the heaviest weight possible while maintaining the speed. Redo the test every week to upgrade the weight.

2. **Maximum Sustainable Power (MSP) workout.** Break the 12 steps into mini-sets and continually increase the weight and duration over time from 1 to 4 minutes while maintaining speed.

35-pounds/2:30 sets. On the bike, SpinScan tests showed that her wattage rose a stunning 28 percent from late 2015 to May 2016, just after her win at Barrio Logan.

"People have taken drugs to get an increase like that," said DeVore.

Fortunately, Mueller had room to keep pushing on the Maximum Overload workouts. Her Bonneville speed record

Raise the weight by 2.5-pound increments. Here is the progression:

1. Start with three 1-minute sets: Break them into 15-second mini-sets.

2. Rest 4 minutes between sets to get full recovery: Do nothing at all or only core and upper-body exercises (pull-ups, planks, pikes, etc.) to rest the legs and lower the heart rate to normal.

3. Push to 2-minute sets: Add 15-second increments to each workout, working up to 2-minute sets. Use the same weight as in the earlier 1-minute sets, with no slowing of your speed.

4. Stay at 2-minute sets and increase your baseline weight: If you do the 2-minute sets comfortably, do another 6-rep baseline weight test. Generally limit the increase to 2.5 pounds or 10 percent.

5. Keep raising your baseline weight until it slows you down: Keep your speed. You must maintain speed to build MSP. Work up to the heaviest weight that you can still maintain your speed. If this was a bike, the weight would be the "right gear."

6. Stretch-out the set to 4 minutes: This is what puts the "sustainable" in MSP.

attempt was still months away at the time, and her coach Howard wanted to raise her MSP further. Since Mueller had already topped out at 35-pound dumbbells (finding that 40-pounders slowed her down too much, while 30-pounders made her no faster), DeVore had her extend her explosive weighted walking lunge sets to 4 minutes to develop more sustained power.

Of course, the deadlift and the explosive weighted walking lunge are not the only exercises used in a Maximum Overload workout. You'll do ab exercises and planks for the core, lat pulls for the back, single-leg presses, squats, and more. Some special mobility exercises will be used to correct imbalances and kyphosis-related postural issues that get in the way of proper form on the strength and power exercises, especially for older riders. To squeeze every watt of power out of your body, there can be no weak link.

Ultimately, however, the deadlift and the explosive weighted walking lunge are the one-two punch that makes this program go. "To make the best use of them," says DeVore, "you gotta understand the physics—know the difference between strength and power. It's the key that unlocks your MSP and potential on the bike."

Maximum Overload Math and Exercise Correlation

You may wonder: Now that you understand the difference between strength and power, what weight do you need to produce the greatest amount of power?

First, let's do the math, which was briefly introduced earlier. Since the goal here is to build the greatest MSP quickly and safely, you should use the heaviest weight you can to move rapidly and under control for 12 walking-lunge steps (i.e., 6 reps), with "failure" reached on the 7th rep. (Failure is the point where the last rep cannot be done with proper form and speed, or at all.)

For example: If you easily do 10 reps with a 15-pound

dumbbell in each hand, that weight is too light. Move up to 17.5- or 20-pounders to bring your maximum reps down to 6 and to maximize your power output.

When done at Absolute Power Output (APO), that heavy weight, moved rapidly, elicits the greatest muscle-fiber recruitment (i.e., it "maximizes" the overload). By contrast, performing 20 or 30 reps of a lighter weight at high speed doesn't allow you to produce your APO, inspiring much less, if any, overloads in muscle recruitment. It's submaximal— just too easy.

"A submaximal output is a waste of time if you are trying to improve your MSP," DeVore says. "You have to lift as heavy a weight as possible with the highest velocity. NOT the heaviest possible weight."

The idea here is to get the body used to performing at APO for as long as possible without going to failure. That replicates what happens on a hard bike effort: You push hard, but at a sustainable pace. If you slip into failure, your ride is over; you're wasted and can't recover quickly enough to keep up with the peloton. The only time you want to go to failure is at the finish line.

Once you establish your 6-reps-to-failure (12 steps) dumbbell weight in the Baseline APO Test, you'll do 6 reps/12 steps of the MSP workout's 3-reps-and-rest mini-sets, as described in the previous section. That'll keep you cool and recovered, allowing you to amass more reps and a bigger overload than you are able to achieve doing the 12-straight-steps plan. Amassing this total overload in power—i.e., your MSP—is where the program's value comes from, as it directly correlates to MSP on the bike.

Over time, your MSP totals will increase through two components: increased workout time and increased weight without any diminishment in movement speed.

After finding your initial baseline APO, your maiden Maximum Overload workout will consist of three 1-minute sets of the prescribed exercise, each set divided into 15-second mini-sets that include 3 reps and rest. As mentioned several times and fully explained a bit later and in Chapter 2, DeVore believes the best do-it-yourself exercise to work the primary mover muscles of cycling is the explosive weighted walking lunge (with thrusters, push presses, wall balls, box jumps, and other leg-centric movements optional). (Note that 1 rep of walking lunges includes two steps—a right and a left. The other exercises use both legs at once.) You don't need to do two different exercises—or have the time to.

As you get fitter, you grow the 1-minute sets into 2-minute sets and eventually top out at 4 minutes. DeVore has found diminishing returns after 4 minutes with Zabriskie and other clients because nonleg parts of the body (shoulders, hands, and lower back) often break down. Including recovery time of about 4 to 6 minutes more or less between the sets, the duration of the entire workout will rise from 11 minutes to 20 minutes as your maximum overload grows. You may find you need more or less recovery time to bring your heart rate down to normal. Remember, to build your biggest MSP, you only want to do Maximum Overload at APO effort, not submaximal effort.

The 2-minute mark is a key threshold. You will stay here a while and raise your baseline weight several times. Get there with your baseline weight by progressing to 1:15, 1:30,

1:45, to 2:00, feeling free to skip directly from 1 minute to 2 minutes if you're fit enough. When you're comfortable working out for 2 minutes, upgrade to a higher baseline weight by doing another 7-rep test to failure, seeing if you can maintain the same velocity at the higher weight. In other words, you don't want to slow down. Generally, raise the weight by 2.5 pounds or not more than 10 percent. So if your initial baseline was a 20-pound dumbbell in each hand, try 22.5-pounders—and remember to keep up the speed. Keep raising the weight until it starts to slow you down. Again, slow, submaximal efforts won't give you MSP. You are training to move faster, not slower.

Cycling provides a good metaphor here. You want to find the dumbbell weight (or gearing) that allows you to move the fastest the longest. If you use too heavy a dumbbell (too big a gear), you'll move (pedal) way too slowly. On the other hand, with too little weight (too low a gear), you spin out. Find the heaviest weight (biggest gear) at which you can maintain your speed (pedal cadence), then start stretching out the workout time.

THE EXERCISES

As Maximum Overload has evolved, DeVore has spent a lot of time searching for exercises that mimic and support the motion of pedaling a bike. He replaced the rare isokinetic machine that Zabriskie used with several do-it-yourself exercises that use easily available dumbbells, barbells, and medicine balls.

The DIY Maximum Overload exercise of choice is the one

that Denise Mueller and most people use, the explosive weighted walking lunge, done with a dumbbell in each hand. Here's why DeVore likes it.

1. It offers similar one-legged biomechanics movement to a pedal stroke, explosively hitting the quads, hamstrings, hips, and lower back (especially if you lean forward in the time-trial position).

2. The movement is easy and safe for anyone to learn and control. Just use the first two steps to establish a rhythm.

3. Dumbbells are everywhere and cheap. You can also do it with bricks, milk cartons, or buckets of paint.

4. It has a low risk of injury. There is no ballistic movement or jumping, so it's safe for joints.

5. It's easy to self-coach and measure the count and velocity. You can tell when you're slowing down or going too fast.

6. It is doable even with bad knees, given the minimal impact. A reverse lunge lessens the impact even more.

Note: There are options if you don't like the explosive weighted walking lunge, including wall balls, thrusters, push presses, kettlebell swings, split squats, and box jumps or step-ups (although this one is potentially dangerous when you fatigue, because you can miss the box or fall off it). They all work similar muscles, but not as well or as conveniently as the explosive weighted walking lunge. And none are single-leg exercises.

The full Maximum Overload workout begins with several

minutes of dynamic warm-up drills. Follow that with several ab exercises, lat pulls, deadlifts, single-leg presses, and more. Using the explosive weighted walking lunge or another power exercise, establish your current APO weight by doing a Baseline APO Test—three sets of 6 reps/12 steps (1 rep = 2 steps). With these two barbells in hand, you then go to the grand finale and signature Maximum Overload measurement device: the Maximum Sustainable Power (MSP) workout. This one is done at a brisk, consistent velocity with 40 to 50 percent less step count (3 to 4 reps/6 to 8 steps) than your baseline. Mueller typically does three 2-minute MSP walking-lunge sets, DeVore's recommendation for everyone with normal biomechanics. As you get fitter, see if you can keep your speed and push the duration to 3 and 4 minutes.

FINALLY, ENJOY THE PSYCHE-UP FACTOR

Not to be overlooked in a discussion of Maximum Overload is the unique sense of motivation, coherency, and organization the program brings to strength training.

This book's coauthor, Roy Wallack, who's been toying with the training since he met DeVore in early 2013, found that the buildup from the body-weight warm-up exercises through the core work, back work, one-legged presses, heavy deadlifts, and finally the grand finale of the day, the explosive walking lunges/MSP workout, almost has a "drumroll" quality to it. "After half an hour of setting the table for the big test, with a mix of dread and anticipation," he says, "you stake out a clear path on the gym floor, grab a couple dumbbells, watch the second hand strike 12, and push off on the walking lunges, totally focused on the next 10 or 15 minutes (three rounds of 2 to 4 minutes each with rest in between) that will give you a 'final score' for the day. It becomes its own competition.

"Frankly, at that moment, knowing these lunges are going to make you faster on your bike is the furthest thing from your mind. You want a PR in the gym right now. And nothing is going to stop you."

Then, on Saturday, you coincidentally find yourself with the same attitude on the bike.

2

THE EXERCISES

Maximum Overload's core-, back-, and leg-blasting exercises will supercharge you on the bike. Here's how to do them right.

You're a cyclist—not a bodybuilder. Your world is wind, sun, a Pinerello, and Lycra spandex—not a dank, musty cave populated by sweaty, grunting, neckless mesomorphs clanking iron. In the gym, you're a geek, an alien, a stranger in a strange land. You know handlebars, not pull-up bars. You clean your chain, not clean and jerk. So it's only natural you'd be a bit confused in the gym environment.

"After years of searching for the lightest possible bike gear, you're telling me that I have to lift heavy weights, the more the better?" you're saying to yourself. And by the way, what's the difference between a barbell and a dumbbell? What's a deadlift? What's a set?

The gym intimidates lots of people—especially skinny bike riders with shaved legs. Yes, maybe you've done a spin class or hopped on an elliptical machine. Maybe you've done a few biceps curls with 15-pound dumbbells and the obligatory core exercises—after all, everyone reading this book will eventually know that weight training is essential for maintaining muscle mass and bone density, issues of particular concern to cyclists (see Chapter 8). But the reality is that most cyclists wouldn't know the difference between a deadlift and a squat and have no idea that a weight-lifting program *done correctly* can help them pedal a bike faster and with Maximum Sustainable Power (MSP).

Done correctly is printed in italics because the sequence and form of the exercises are essential to progress and reducing injury risk. You don't want to get hurt or waste your time in the gym. So this chapter will give you the 30,000-foot overview of how and why the basic Maximum Overload workout is structured as it is, why certain exercises were chosen, the importance of their order, and step-by-step tutorials of how to execute them safely and effectively. Extra exercises are provided for those who may need easier options initially or have limitations. We wait until Chapter 4 to give you the numbers—the reps, sets, times and progressions of the workout program over a season.

The Maximum Overload workout has five exercise sections, which roll out in the following order:

I. Dynamic Warm-Up Exercises/Movement Prep

II. Core/Mobility and Upper-Body Strength Exercises

III. Lower-Body Strength Exercises

IV. Lower-Body Power Exercises and the Absolute Power Output (APO) Test. The latter, done with two 12-step walking lunges, lets you check to see if you have progressed to a new, higher benchmark weight. Done on a Wednesday, it will not tire you for a hard ride on Saturday.

V. Long-Duration Maximum Sustainable Power (MSP) workout. The ultimate goal of the Maximum Overload program, MSP allows you to push the workout longer. Done on a Monday, it allows plenty of recovery time for rides later in the week and on the weekend.

The workout proceeds in this sequence to build up safely to a dramatic, session-ending MSP workout with a power exercise like an explosive walking lunge. Everything you do is focused on getting your body 100 percent primed for power, for setting a new MSP personal record.

It starts with an extensive dynamic warm-up for mobility and movement prep, moves to exercises that activate the core and back, then homes in on primary-mover exercises (hips, quads, and posterior chain) that target pure strength, such as deadlifts and single-leg presses (for equivalent power in each leg). Only then, with the joints lubed, the blood flowing, the neuromuscular pathways humming, the stretch-shortening cycle primed, are you ready to hammer your muscles with strength and speed at all once—meaning you will be developing power with power exercises like the preferred explosive walking lunge.

Warning: Don't shortcut the warm-up! An extensive warm-up is so necessary for safety and performance that pro athletes will routinely take 45 minutes just to execute a warm-up—which is as long as we might spend during an entire Maximum Overload workout.

Of course, the pros have all day to work out and follow up with massage, ultrasound, and cryotherapy. Working out is their full-time job. It's Jacques DeVore's job to get you safely through a 40- to- 60-minute Maximum Overload workout that fits in your life. Safety comes first, and it is simply unsafe to forget the warm-up and the preliminary core/mobility and upper-body exercises. Think about it: Would you do an all-out sprint the minute you unrack your bike? Never! That's a prescription for pulled muscles and aching joints. For the same reason, quads, glutes, hamstrings, and your entire body won't react well to heavy deadlifts and explosive weighted walking lunges done the minute you saunter into your local 24 Hour Fitness. So don't waste your time. To get the most out of your muscles, warm them up. If you are short on time, do a lower quantity of the exercises, but do some from each group, in the prescribed order, to prepare for the final MSP workout.

Beyond the warm-up, a key long-term goal of the overall Maximum Overload workout is to build the superstructure to support your new stronger legs. Leg power can't be developed in isolation, even in a leg-centric sport like cycling. The whole body is a unit, with legs, core, arms, and the upper body all connected with the bike.

It's not that the upper body and the hands provide any power to the pedals per se. But they give the legs the connection to the core platform to leverage off and produce full power. If the kinetic chain (the linkage of bones and muscles) from handlebar to pedals is broken or weak, you can't tap all your potential power.

To illustrate this, DeVore loves to speculate on what would happen if he was racing against superstar sprinter Mark Cavendish in a 100-meter sprint. There's one condition, however: The Englishman must take his hands off the handlebars and only use his legs. "Chances are he couldn't keep up with me," says DeVore, who's old enough to be Cavendish's father.

This is why, after the dynamic warm-up, the Maximum Overload workout hits the core and upper body. Only after this does it get to the legs' heavy strength exercises (such as the deadlift), and finally to the high-velocity power exercises (such as explosive walking lunges).

REMINDER: START WITH A SELF-ASSESSMENT

Before you begin the Maximum Overload program, you need to do a self-assessment. Everyone has weaknesses, imbalances, and mobility limitations that get worse with age and injuries. Cyclists over age 50, with years in the hunched-over riding position exacerbating a lifetime of sitting at a desk, may be shocked by their hip, knee, and thoracic spine immobility and postural degradation. If these issues aren't identified and addressed up front, you not only won't get the full benefit of Maximum Overload's heavy weight lifting and power training, but you also will probably get injured.

For example: Despite a monster aerobic system that

allows him to stay with and sometimes beat men 20 or 30 years younger, 68-year-old John Howard had so many mobility issues that DeVore determined that it was too risky for him to jump into the standard Maximum Overload workout without additional exercises. Like many longtime cyclists, Howard has a pronounced degree of kyphosis, a slumping posture with rounded-forward shoulders and upper back that is caused by both natural aging and by cycling's unusual leaned-forward position. Lifting heavy weights with this posture is a recipe for a strained/injured thoracic spine, lower back, and a lot more. DeVore saw the problem as soon as Howard began the dynamic warm-up. While doing a lunge, his thoracic spine and hip mobility was so limited that he couldn't get his hips down or elevate an arm simultaneously, which limited his ability to do all the exercises of the full Maximum Overload workout.

After just a few minutes of special mobility drills, Howard's before-and-after postures showed a profound improvement, allowing him to tiptoe into lifting heavier weights. Still, DeVore expressly warned him away from the higher weights being used by Mueller, who is 25 years younger and had some strength-training background and excellent mobility. To strengthen Howard in a risk-free manner, DeVore gave Howard more mobility drills (see Chapter 3) and prescribed more use of the single-leg press than the deadlift. "Sometimes you have to take a step backward to make a giant leap forward," he says.

DeVore sees a lot of cyclists with big cardio engines and battered bodies. He calls them "horribly fit."

"Plenty of people can throw their feet over the top tube

and ride 50 miles," he says. "But it's like driving on the freeway with bald tires. Yes, you can go 90 mph; just hope you don't hit a pothole, because then you're screwed."

Continuing the car analogy, DeVore notes that tires are "rated" for a reason. "As the speed gets higher, going too fast will rip the tire apart," he says. "Put an economy tire on a Lamborghini, and you're done. It'll self-destruct." The lesson: If you make your legs stronger, you have to fix and build the rest of your body to match the higher performance they can give you.

Again, you absolutely must do a self-assessment before you jump into Maximum Overload. Recognizing that kyphosis and mobility limitations are major issues for cyclists and that everyone has different biomechanical issues to work around, we have devoted the next chapter, Chapter 3, entirely to a self-assessment checklist and special mitigating exercises and drills. We recommend that everyone read Chapter 3 to find out where they stand before jumping into the Maximum Overload exercises described here.

EXERCISE TUTORIALS

Important: Do the exercises correctly to maximize safety and effectiveness.

The exercises used in the Maximum Overload program have been chosen for effectiveness and practicality. They're doable at any gym with standard gym equipment. You don't need the rare isokinetic machine on which DeVore trained Dave Zabriskie or the VersaPulley, the rower-like "inertial-power" training machine that Denise Mueller and John Howard used several times in DeVore's gym in West LA. In fact, Mueller and Howard did nearly all their workouts back home in Encinitas, using the standard equipment found at their homes and local gyms: dumbbells, barbells, inflatable exercise balls, towel core slides, pull-up bars, and lat-pull and leg-press machines.

Don't forget that the whole point of the Maximum Overload workout is a buildup to each session's grand finale: the MSP workout. The drumroll starts slowly with the dynamic warm-up, progresses through the core and upper-body exercises, builds through the lower-body strength exercises, and explodes in the lower-body power exercises. Whether you do the workout alone or with a partner, it is highly motivating to end a workout with a test that not only gives you metrics you can compare to previous workouts, but that you know will make you a more functional person and a better bike rider.

A final note: Put safety first. Make sure you're constantly checking in with yourself—that all systems are go. If you hurt, it's a warning to stop, take a step back, lessen the weight or the reps, or lower the intensity. If you are hesitant, lighten it up. When you get comfortable, raise the weight on the next round.

I. Dynamic Warm-Up

Whatever you don't do, you're not in shape for.

"'But I'm fit!' they say, and then they can't do three lunges in a row," says DeVore. "Lunges aren't difficult, but require some body stabilization as well as strength and power. People get one-dimensional in their fitness." Being able to push two pedals in a linear circle all day long does not prepare you to squat low and shuffle from side to side for 10 seconds or to deadlift 100 pounds. To get your body ready to move in all dimensions in complex multijoint exercises under load, as you'll be doing in Maximum Overload, you need to prep it with a warm-up.

The dynamic warm-up drills listed here, typically each done in 6 to 10 steps up and back in a hallway at a leisurely pace (1 to 5 seconds per step) and completed in about 10 minutes by experienced people, do several good things: Raise heart rate; activate muscles, tendons, and ligaments; lubricate and mobilize joints, especially the knees, hips, ankles, and shoulders; and initiate neuromuscular firing, so your muscles will be primed to move heavy loads. Studies have found that old-fashioned lie-on-the-floor static stretching reduces your ability to produce power, which is why sophisticated sports teams and individual athletes have all gone to dynamic warm-ups.

Important: **Do these in the order listed.** The level of muscle activation and intensity increases through the series.

Using only body-weight exercises that can be performed anywhere, the dynamic warm-up also provides a valuable step-by-step check-in. It can tell you, "Is my body A-okay?" If odd aches and pains arise during the warm-up, it may be an indication that something is amiss. You'll need to dial back the intensity until the pain goes away or stop the exercise. Pain is your "Houston, we have a problem." If it persists, scrub the launch. If it hurts, don't do it. Figure it out before you proceed further, so you don't hurt it more.

There are hundreds of dynamic warm-up exercises in the fitness world. Some are more shoulder-driven, some hip-driven. DeVore has selected the exercises that can be done in the least amount of time with maximum effectiveness. The warm-up makes a gradual progression in mobility and heart rate, culminating with explosive skipping.

Warm-up rates vary for everyone. Generally, as you get older, the warm-up needs to be longer. Some people are so out of shape regardless of age that the dynamic warm-up *is* the workout. If that's the case for you, focus on form, put your heart into it, and do it over and over again until you feel ready to move on to the rest of the program. You can progress fast once you can execute the warm-up effectively, so do not be discouraged.

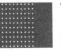

Walking Lunge with Thoracic Spine-Mobility Twist

Pause in the middle of a long forward lunge step, stepping out with your left leg first, and put your hands on the ground inside your forward leg. Then plant your left hand on the floor inside of your left leg and twist your torso to the right so that it is perpendicular to the floor, look at the sky, and reach up straight up with your right hand. Your left hand stays on the floor, helping you balance. Then step forward and do the same thing on the left. This mobilizes the hips; engages the hamstrings, ribcage, and hip joint; and opens up the shoulders/thoracic spine.

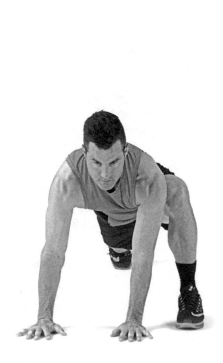
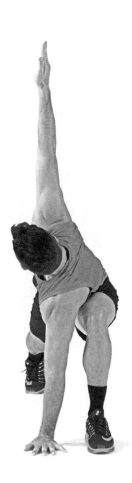

Sidestep Hip Mobility Lunge with Arms Up

Lunge to the side while you keep your head and back up, raise your arms to the sky, and sit deep into the lunge sideways. This furthers the unslumping of your upper back, mobilizes and activates the hips, and works the adductors and the gluteus medius and gluteus minimus, which give you the lateral strength to help keep your hips stabilized. The motion of cycling does not significantly work these muscles, yet they are important for keeping an efficient pistonlike pedal stroke and maintaining hip stability for your weight lifting at the gym.

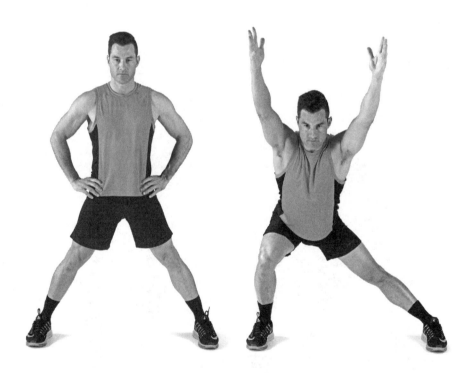

Stretch-Band Lateral Side Shuffle

Place a stretch band around your ankles and another above your knees and do a lateral sidestep lunge in the squatted position, keeping your hands down. This further activates the hip muscles, blasting the important but underworked abductors and the gluteus medius and minimus. There are different levels of band resistance. Use one that allows you to shuffle about 15 yards and back.

If you don't have access to the inexpensive stretch bands, the body-weight hip thrust/glute bridge (see page 63) is a good hip activation/warm-up.

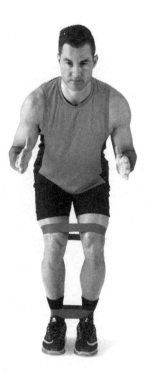
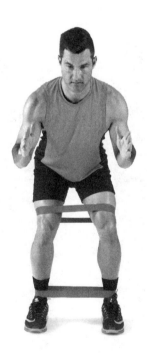

Cowboy Walk

With the stretch bands still in place, walk forward while moving your legs in an in-to-out pattern. You'll look like a drunken cowboy with six guns on. This continues to work the lateral stabilizer muscles and hip flexors while transitioning you back to forward movement.

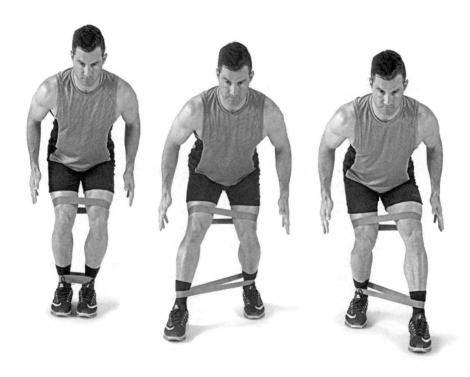

Hip Thrust/ Glute Bridge

Lying flat on your back, bend your legs at 45 degrees and spread your arms out to the side for stability. Keeping your core tight, push your butt up into the bridge position. Focus on squeezing your glutes, keeping them flexed and your back straight the whole time (a 1- to 5-second hold). This is very effective when using a bench to support your shoulders and arms. As you get stronger, you can go to a single-leg bridge or add weight to either the double- or single-leg exercise by putting a plate or dumbbell on your stomach or by wearing a weighted vest.

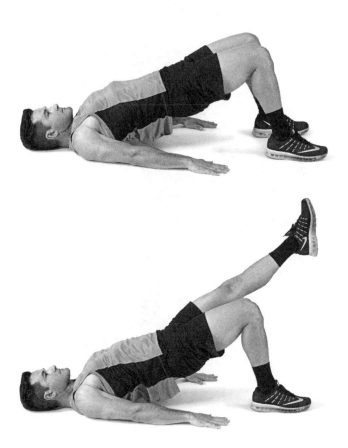

High-Knee
Skip

This fun, high-energy, explosive movement not only makes you feel 10 again, but also activates the stretch-shortening reflex, rockets the heart rate, and primes the neuromuscular firing of the quads and glutes. Jump as high as possible.

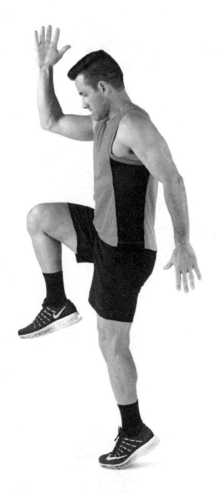

II. Core Strength and Upper-Body Exercises

All the muscles between the hands and feet have an impact on performance. If any of them are weak or injured, the kinetic chain is broken or compromised. For example: If your hips are weak, you'll have problems with your lower back—the latter will try to compensate for the former. Your weakest link may not cause problems in a short event, but as distances grow, so will the strain. Everything might be hunky-dory until mile 85, when the shoulders and neck start to ache, remnants of that old injury from high school. That ache eventually slows you down. Your weak points always come out of the blue to bite you in the 11th hour of endurance events. So don't let them be weak; work on your known weak links and your general mobility. It'll allow you to maintain good form and power late in the game.

Even if you lack weak spots, keep in mind that you need to activate all your muscles in the warm-up to support the heavy lower-body strength and power exercises to come.

Core Strength Exercises

A Maximum Overload workout hits the entire core. The reverse hyper lower-back strengthener, done on a rarely seen machine (of course, found at DeVore's gym), can be somewhat replicated by use of a similar do-it-yourself movement done on an inflatable physio ball. A variety of core exercises, including planks, towel slides, and AbDolly rollouts, work the lower-back muscles and the abs in both a static and a dynamic fashion. That's important because stability and mobility together produce human movement.

Reverse Hyper

Two versions: Machine and Physio Ball

Machine Reverse Hypers: Turn yourself into a human reverse-jackknife as you move from a 90-degree-angle torso-to-legs to a straight line, forcing your butt and lower back into action.

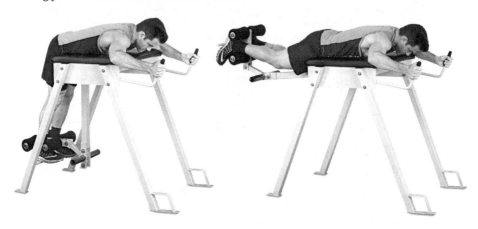

Physio Ball Reverse Hypers: Drape yourself, facedown, over the inflatable ball with your hands and forearms flat on the floor on one side and your feet down on the other. Throw your legs up in the air as high as they'll go, ideally holding them momentarily in place overhead by squeezing/contracting the lower back and glutes.

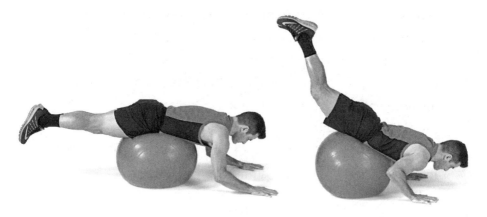

Static Plank and Pelvic-Tilt Plank

Similar to the upper position of a push-up, except that you are resting on your forearms and elbows, the plank blasts both sides of the core if you activate your butt. Hold for a minute.

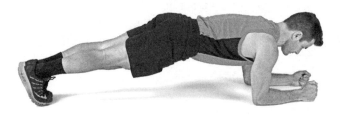

For the pelvic-tilt version, move your elbows 4 to 5 inches ahead of a normal plank, then squeeze everything together as hard as you can, trying to curl your toes and elbows together—like a cat—without actually moving. Done right, you'll begin to shake after 10 seconds (unlike a regular plank, which you can often hold for several minutes). Hold for 30 seconds.

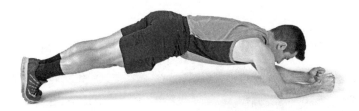

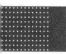

AbDolly Rollout and Body Saw

(Towel slides or ball rolls)

Place your forearms on the dolly and roll forward. Roll out farther little by little as you get stronger, ultimately aiming for a full straight-arm "Superman" position. (Don't push it; Superman is an advanced position that could injure the untrained.) If you don't have an ab-rolling device, use a towel that you don't mind getting dirty and do a body saw: Place your feet on the towel, plant your forearms in place, then slide your feet backward on the floor on the towel (or, in its place, a medicine ball). Hold for a few seconds at the farthest extent, then pull yourself directly forward or raise your butt up into a pike position. Since it works your core in each direction, it strengthens you fast.

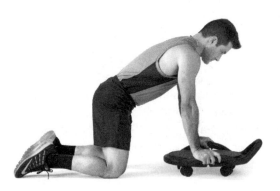

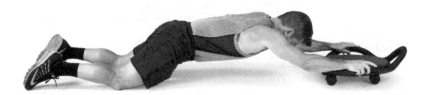

Upper-Body Exercises

On the surface, the upper body doesn't seem to do much in cycling, but it cannot be ignored. After all, you do pull on the handlebar with your hands, and since your hands and feet are contralaterally linked, you can't allow the pulling muscles of the upper body to be weak links. Pulling exercises are often ignored by gym-goers because they work muscles located somewhere you can't see—the back. Cyclists who come into DeVore's gym often have never done a single pull-up—and actually can't do one. That will change rapidly as you do these.

You don't have to do all four of these exercises. Do the push-ups and alternate the pulling exercises.

Bent-Over Dumbbell Row with or without a Bench

When you bend over at the waist, supported by one hand on a bench, and pull a dumbbell to your horizontal torso, it looks suspiciously like your standing position for a sprint. This exercise is hard—and great for rotational, core, and back strength. Start with very light weight.

For a more advanced version, do a bench-free free row, in which you just bend at the waist (with one foot forward and the other back) and row with one arm, holding that position with pure core strength. Engaging your core and back like this is very good for sprinting, as you are pulling across your body, one side then the other. Core strength is really key in the "jump," the first four or five pedal strokes in a sprint. (Once you're up to full speed, the huge power is not involved.)

You'll really notice your core working hard on the bike during steep, out-of-the-saddle climbing in which you've run out of gears or are using a single-speed mountain bike. You're pulling with your hands and driving so hard with your feet that you feel like you're going to rip the handlebars off. That hand-feet connection is total core.

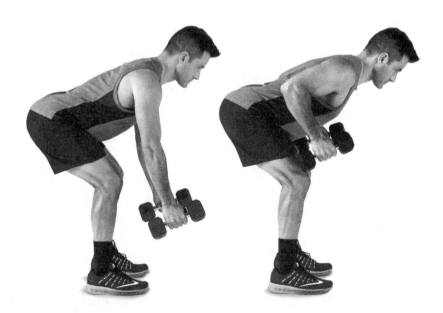

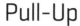

Pull-Up

Maybe the world's most doable, practical, good-for-you exercise, the pull-up is as simple as they get and more beneficial for your all-body health than anything save a body-weight squat. In fact, those two, along with a plank, work everything from head to toe. Cyclists often can't do one pull-up.

To build up to a pull-up, those who are very weak have four options:

1. Use a rubber pull-up assist band.
2. Do lat pulldowns (next exercise).
3. Jump up to the bar and slowly lower yourself. Over time, slow the descent and even start reversing direction.
4. Find a low bar that allows you to keep your feet on the ground or use TRX straps. This way, you control your body angle and the effective amount of body weight lifted.

As you get stronger, move into a more vertical position, i.e., make the pull-ups more vertical. The more upright you become, the more difficult the pull-up becomes. Pull-ups are better to do on rings or with handles that can rotate, as people find that pull-ups can often aggravate the elbows.

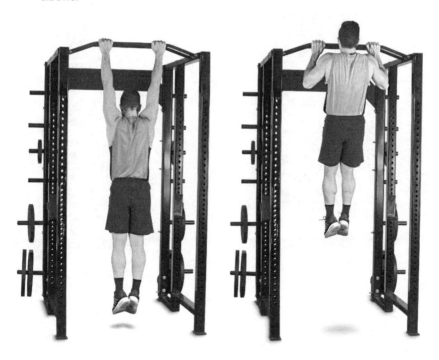

Lat Pulldown

Done on dedicated machines found at every gym in the world, this back strengthener is safe, adjustable, measurable, and easier to start on than a full-blown pull-up. Close-grip overhead lat pulls, which are similar to your position on the bike, are also very helpful in teaching you to retract your scapulas to counteract the rounded-forward kyphosis that is so prevalent among cyclists. Protect your shoulders by keeping your hands in the elbows-in hammer position.

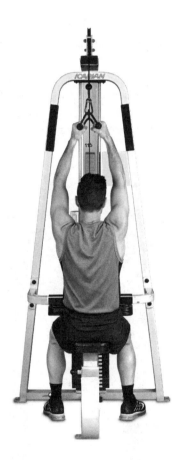
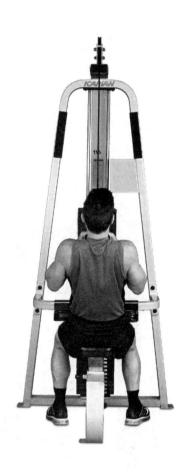

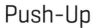

Push-Up

Surprised to see this one? Well, cyclists need some functional shoulder stability/mobility, as well as some upper-body strength for vanity—so you don't look like you're just out of a POW camp. Rule of thumb: If you can't do 10 to 15 reps, you need some work.

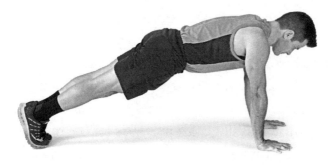

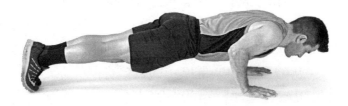

III. Lower-Body Strength Exercises:
The Key to Maximum Overload

Now it's time to get to the nitty-gritty, the meat and potatoes of the Maximum Overload program: strengthening the lower-body muscles that move a biker's body, where your power grid is produced. After all, you don't win a bike race doing 20 pull-ups or walking on your hands.

Keep in mind: These are higher-risk exercises. They are the most important. They use much heavier weight. They must be done correctly and they require a lot more explanation up front. You must know the why and the what.

Warning: Don't do all of these exercises in one workout— you'll be fried. Do 2 to 4 in any one workout. Include one or all of the three foundational exercises: the hex-bar deadlift, Romanian deadlift, and single-leg press. As for the remaining three, mix and match based on your strengths and weaknesses.

As you know by now, high-force strength activities give you the raw force/pushing power you need on the bike, but not the velocity that will produce Maximum Sustainable Power (MSP). They do, however, make the power exercises that follow them better by warming them up and grooving the neuromuscular pathways. (Technically, this is known as Post-Activation Potentiation, or PAP, which we will also put to use with interval training in Chapter 6.)

As mentioned at length in Chapter 1, Maximum Overload's number-one strength exercise is the deadlift, because it allows you to lift very heavy weights safely from a dead stop. That requires a rapid force production that makes it a superb builder of strength, a necessary component of developing power in athletes. The dead stop in the deadlift eliminates the stretch-shortening cycle, the rubber-band effect that helps you spring the weight back up (found in a squat and other exercises). Without that helpful bounce, it's more like a train slowly starting up: You're not going fast initially, but the high-speed force production required to get it going is immense. Also, the deadlift activates the core well and is safe for solo workouts, because when you get tired, you can just drop the weights. That is not the case with a squat, in which your body gets in the way (numerous examples of this failure can be found on YouTube). For that reason, squats are safer when done with a partner.

Also, Maximum Overload uses deadlifts but not squats for an important cycling-functional reason: The deadlift replicates the biomechanical patterning of the pedaling movement and cycling positioning much better than a deep squat does. A cyclist never squats that deep on the bike.

Maximum Overload uses two types of deadlifts: the trap bar and the Romanian. The trap bar deadlift works the quads, glutes, and hamstrings almost as well as a regular straight bar deadlift, but is safer for the lower back. If you can't find a trap bar (it is rare), this exercise can be done with dumbbells and is easier to learn, particularly in clearing your shins. The Romanian deadlift, an entirely different exercise, primarily targets the high hamstrings and glutes, making it a good warm-up for the walking lunge. (You'll feel them when you get out of the car the next day.)

Hex/Trap Bar Deadlift and Dumbbell Deadlift

Why: Use of a hex bar or dumbbells provides less risk of injury to the back than a regular deadlift because the weight is located along the center line of your body. Hip activation in the sim-squatted dumbbell starting position is excellent and very close to the biomechanics of cycling. Be aware that hex bars are not found in most gyms, so you will most likely do this exercise with a dumbbell in each hand, which replicates the hex-bar position. If you insist on doing the deadlift with a conventional straight barbell, watch your back. As the bar must clear your knee, it can re-distribute the weight forward of your center line, stressing the back. Reduce this risk by focusing on getting the hips forward and knees back quickly.

What it works: Glutes, quads and hamstrings, and lower back

• • • • • • • •

Start: With your hands holding the bar or dumbbells, lower your hips, look forward with your head and chin as they are slightly tucked into your chest (known as "packing the neck"), and keep your chest up. Ideal position: If you had a logo on your T-shirt, someone could read it while standing in front of you.

Motion: Stand up by driving through your heels and midfoot into the floor as you rise up, straightening your hips and knees. (Pretend there is a glass wall in front of you that you can't touch, that'll force you to push your hips back and not let your knees break through it.) Do not round your back. Do not use your arms. After standing tall at the finish, reverse the motion and lower the weight back to the ground under control.

Note: The first rep and the last reps carry the most risk, so pay attention to your form. The rep count for this and all the exercises can be found in the workouts in Chapter 4.

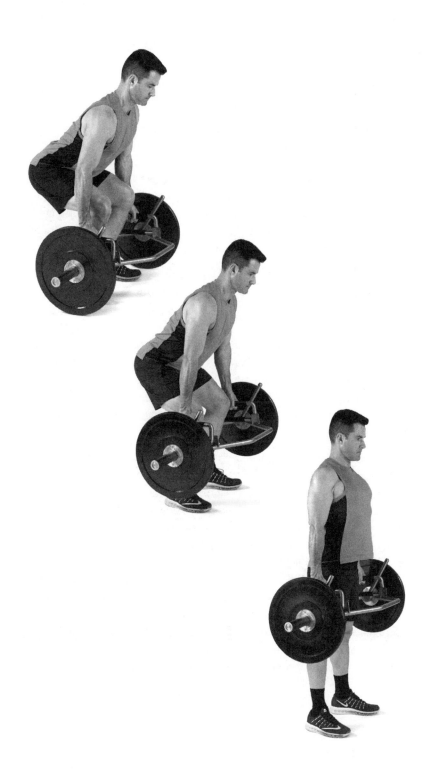

Romanian Deadlift

Why: An excellent glute-hamstring–specific exercise for cyclists, the Romanian deadlift addresses the hamstrings, which are not the primary focus in some of the other exercises, and preps you for the stretch-shortening cycle used in the lunges. If your hamstrings are weak, they can't decelerate as well to control the speed, then transition back into acceleration. (A lot of knee injuries come from trying to decelerate on weak hamstrings and glutes, which puts all the load on the knees.) Strong hamstrings are great for climbing out of the saddle (because you're pulling up) and are what allow you to "stick the landing" on a jump.

What it works: Hamstrings and glutes, with lower back and abdominals

· · · · · · · ·

Start: Usually set up with much less than half the weight of a regular deadlift, stand with your feet shoulder-width apart, and hold the bar or dumbbells at hip level with a pronated (your palms facing down) grip. Position your shoulders back, with your back arched or flat and your knees slightly bent. Again, typically your maximum lift weights may be less than half of a regular deadlift.

Motion: Lower the bar by moving your hips/butt back as far as you can—with a slight bend of your legs. Keep the bar moving as close to your body and legs as possible, with your head looking forward and your shoulders back. Stop when the bar is about mid-shin, below your knee; further movement may risk back strain. At the bottom of your range of motion, squeeze hard on your glutes and return to the starting position by driving your hips forward to stand straight up.

Practice the Romanian deadlift without a bar by squatting, touching your fingertips to the floor, and keeping them there while elevating your hips and pushing your butt back. All the while, don't straighten your legs. You'll feel it loading your hamstrings. Once in that position, hinge at your waist while keeping your back flat and slightly arched and then rise up to standing. This is the movement you are looking for under load.

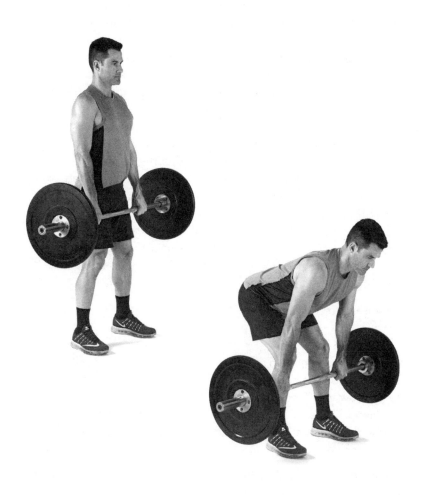

Single-Leg Press

Why: It identifies and fixes leg-strength imbalances. Typically you have a dominant leg; the single-leg press helps you develop the nondominant side. On a bike, equalizing the two legs can provide a huge performance boost, since they share the load. Even a slight 49/51 imbalance between the two makes for a big difference over a long day. In bike-racer parlance, bringing the weak leg's strength up to the other one adds more "domestiques" (muscle fibers) to your power supply.

While the double-leg press can be used as a lightweight warm-up for the single-leg press, it is easy to do wrong and can lead to lower-back injuries. DeVore does not like double-leg presses for this reason.

The single-leg press has two other things going for it: It's good for cyclists and older folk with weak upper bodies who may have trouble doing a heavy deadlift, which requires grip strength, back strength, and T-spine strength and mobility. This is why John Howard used single-leg presses to build up his legs while his T-spine mobility problem was being fixed. Also, the single-leg press does a great job of activating the quads, one of cycling's prime movers.

What it works: Quadriceps, with glutes and hamstrings

· · · · · · · ·

Start: First, warm up with lightweight two-legged presses. Then, switch to one leg (just take one foot off), placing your other foot on the ground. Do not move your foot under the load as you will risk injuring your knee. Keeping your head and chest up, push to the point of a slight knee bend— don't lock out. Push through your heel. Make sure your hips are pinned to the pad and do not roll up.

Motion: Starting in the leg-extended position after a two-leg push, bend your hip and knee. Don't move your pelvis and arch your lower back to help manage the load; flexing or rounding the back risks hurting it.

Keep your back as flat as possible against the pad. Pin your butt to the pad; don't let it roll up. Adjust your foot position or lower the weight until you can do it without rolling your butt. Slowly lower the weight as far as you can; don't speed through it, as going too fast may risk a rib injury, since your quad presses into your rib cage. Don't get lazy and rush it; the single-leg press is better done slowly than fast. Pause briefly at the bottom of your range of motion, then push, extending your knees and hip as you return to the starting position. Do not lock out your knees.

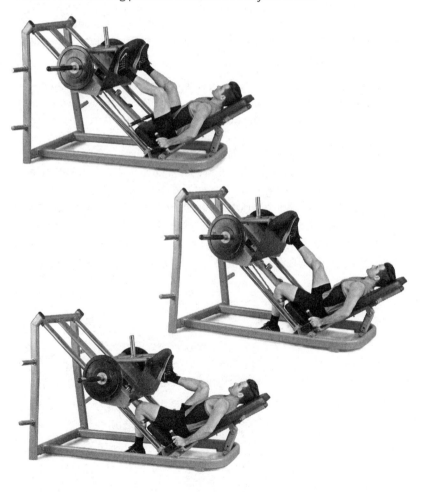

Reaching Lunge

Why: This cycling-specific exercise, which puts your body in a time-trial–like position, is a very good unilateral strength exercise. The reaching aspect works the glutes better than a normal lunge, which is more quad-dominant.

What it works: Glutes, quads, hamstrings, and some core

· · · · · · · ·

Start: Facing forward, place one foot on the back end of slide board and the other on the concrete in front of the board. Keep your front knee over your heel. If at home, place your front foot on the kitchen floor, and your back foot on a towel.

Motion: Simultaneously slide your back leg to the rear as you reach forward with your hands and imagine touching the floor in front of you. Keep your back flat and hinge at the waist. (You won't be able to reach the floor, as you will run into the quad). Over time, as your rear leg reaches farther back, you'll be able to lean your chest forward so that it rests on top of your front-leg quad, with your chin on your knee and your arms reaching way out in front—keeping your back flat and hinged at the waist. Try it unweighted at first, then do it while holding light weights in your hands. Whatever you do, don't pull your arms back—that makes it too easy to slide the leg back. Increase the weight by holding a dumbbell once you can easily keep your arms out.

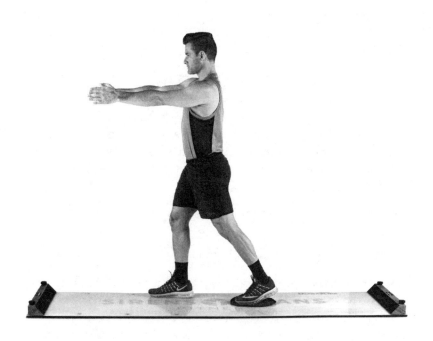

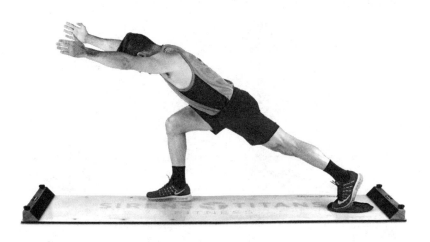

Bulgarian Split Squat

Why: Working one leg at a time helps correct lower-body muscle and strength imbalances. The Bulgarian's elevated rear leg, which allows you to drop the front hip and build strong glutes, does not stress the lower back like a traditional back squat can. It's also very safe if you are lifting by yourself; just drop the dumbbells. And it's easier than regular squats for those with limited shoulder mobility or wrist issues (which a lot of cyclists have due to frequent crashes).

What it works: Glutes, like a regular squat plus knee stability (because it's unilateral)

. . . .

Start: Assume a lunge-type position with your back leg up on a bench or a small plyo box. Start with a low-height box or a step—2 or 3 inches high. (You'll need lots of hip flexor mobility to do it if your back leg is too high—go no higher than 12 to 18 inches.) Hold a dumbbell in each hand and keep your head and back erect.

Motion: Drop your body 12 inches or more, bending at your front knee while keeping your back vertical. Sit back into the bench as you lower in order to continue sitting up tall, then push through your front heel and come up. DeVore likes to see the hip go just below parallel.

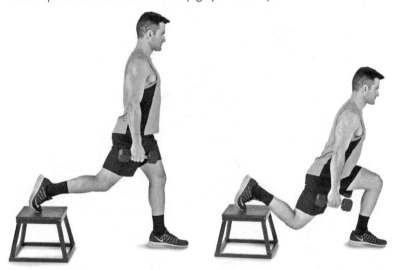

IV. Lower-Body Power Exercises

As you recall, power and strength are different. Power has a velocity component, an explosion that moves the muscle quickly. Power is the culmination of the Maximum Overload program, the boost that gives you your goal of maximum sustainable power.

While the Maximum Overload Absolute Power Output (APO) test and Maximum Sustainable Power (MSP) workout is done with explosive walking lunges, which do the best job of replicating the muscular movements and power used in cycling, several other lower-body power exercises are useful for the sake of variety. These others can help prepare the body for the lunges or substitute for them, providing weight-lifting rookies and veterans some options.

Having several power exercises allows for a quick substitute if a knee problem flares up when you do lunges. Wall balls, which use lightweight medicine balls, provide good entry points and a progression for beginners. Moderately deep push presses/thrusters and single-leg crossover plyo-box step-jumps can provide much of the benefit of the lunges.

In order of our preference, lunges are the clear number one as a do-it-yourself cycling-specific power exercise. If all you have are dumbbells and the walking room for six consecutive steps, nothing else comes close.

Explosive Walking Lunge

Why: Superb for cycling because it hits all the primary mover muscles, especially the quads and glutes, with fairly heavy overload in an alternating, unilateral leg activity. It also works core rotational stability. Lunges are a closed-chain, multijoint, compound exercise that maximizes the sustained power development when you make them "explosive"—done by leaning forward and blasting out of each long step. The leaning forward, hinging-at-the-waist aspect, a subtle change from a standard walking lunge, gets greater hip engagement.

What it works: Quadriceps, glutes, calves, and hamstrings

· · · · · · · ·

Start: Stand with your feet shoulder-width apart and dumbbells in each hand. (You can start off just with body weight, depending on your level of strength and power. If you are a heavier cyclist, you may not need dumbbells to start. Your body weight serves as a built-in dumbbell.)

Motion: Step forward with your right leg, bending at a 90-degree angle at your knee and dropping down until your rear (left) knee nearly touches the ground. Keep your back straight with a forward lean and your front (right) knee in a vertical line with your front foot. Without pausing, drive forward through your front foot in your heel and midfoot, bringing your left foot to the front position, maintaining an upright-lean torso throughout—and immediately drive through into the next step without stopping. Flow over the top; don't put your left foot down. If you have a hard time keeping your balance, take a wider step until you get comfortable with the exercise.

Be mindful of your speed while doing the walking lunge. If you are sprinting, the weight is too light. If you are lurching through slowly, it's too heavy. Find a moderately heavy weight you can maintain a good pace with. Your goal is to develop power, and that is done through both overload and speed.

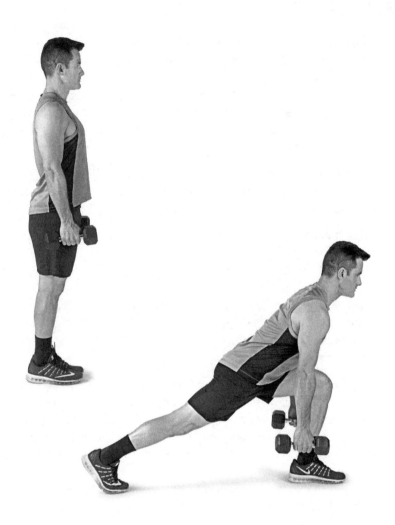

"Deep" Push Press/ Thruster

Why: The push press melds a partial squat with a minimal overhead press, hitting all the primary cycling mover muscles and incorporating the stretch-reflex cycle for MSP. Convenient and doable anywhere, it's executed with a quick hip explosion that floats a pair of dumbbells, a barbell, one or two kettlebells, or other found objects overhead. DeVore favors dumbbells over a barbell because they are easier and better for improving shoulder stability.

Note: A "deep" push press adds more depth to the slight knee dip/quad explosion of a regular push press. A thruster is essentially a deeper version of a push press.

What it works: Quads, with glutes, hamstrings, middle back, shoulders, traps, and triceps

· · · · · · · ·

Start: With your hands holding the bar or dumbbells about shoulder width in the "rack" position (top of your front deltoids, pushing into your clavicles, and lightly touching your throat), drop into a partial squat, pushing your hips and butt back.

Motion: Partially squatted, with your knees below your hips, inhale as you prepare to blast upward. Explode through your heels as your legs straighten. Done correctly, your feet will actually leave the ground. Accelerating as you reach full standing position, hold the bar tight with your fingers as the momentum carries the weight toward the ceiling and lock your legs. The bar should terminate at the end of your fully extended arms with little or no arm effort. Lock out your arms at the top, maintaining tightness from head to toe. Then drop the weight to the rack position, descend back into a partial squat, and do it again.

Note: While there is not a way to accurately measure power on a push press, you can roughly gauge it by keeping track of your speed. If your feet no longer leave the ground, it means your power is diminishing. When your arm effort on the overhead portion becomes too great, it's another sign that leg power is waning and you need to shut down. Don't round your back or let the bar get too far away from your body.

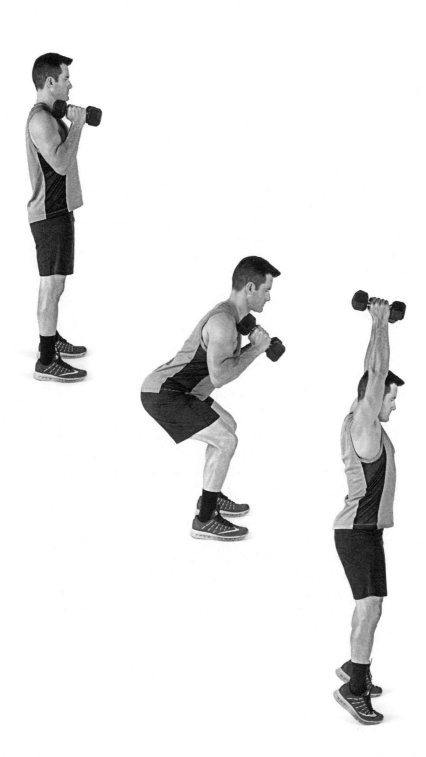

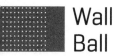

Wall
Ball

Why: Resembling a thruster done with a medicine ball, the wall ball taps the cycling primary mover muscles as you squat down, explode up, and throw a medicine ball to strike a target high on the wall. The exercise has minimal injury risk, as long as you are careful not to curve your lower back as you catch the ball and let its weight pull you forward. Wall ball can be a warm-up or a main exercise. Its power output is easy to measure by the height and accuracy of your throws. As with the push press, focus on propelling the ball with your leg explosion and not with the throw. To fully protect your back, let the ball drop to the ground after each throw.

What it works: Quads, with glutes, hamstrings, middle back, shoulders, traps, and triceps

· · · · · · · ·

Start: Stand 2 feet from the wall with your chest high, your shoulders back, with the ball held at chest height.

Motion: Descend into a half to full squat (with your thighs parallel to the floor or less), then stand up explosively by driving through your heels and snapping at your hips to generate maximum power. On the way up, simultaneously push the ball overhead (it requires more shoulders than the thruster). Released at full standing position with your arms up, note the height of your maximum throw and try to match that each time. (If you're going too high, get a heavier ball.) Most of the ball's movement should come from your hips unweighting it, not your arms.

As the ball returns, receive it in a standing position with a palms-up basket catch with your fingers facing the wall. As you let the weight and momentum pull you back down in into the squat, rotate your palms and fingers outward to facilitate pushing.

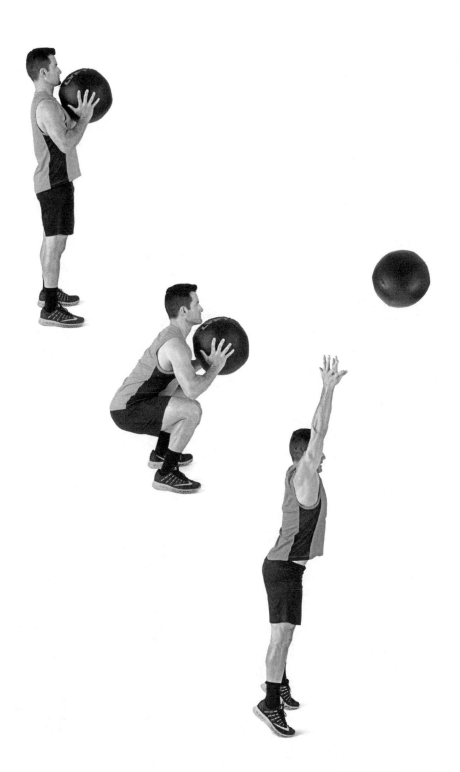

Single-Leg Crossover Plyo Bench Jump

Why: A great unilateral explosive power-producing exercise, these step-ups take you laterally back and forth over a bench. It's safer and more cycling-specific than a box jump, as it works one leg at a time, minimizes the potential of catastrophic falls, and thoroughly works your legs and core.

What it works: Quads, glutes, core, and coordination (Done right, you'll look like you're ready for *Dancing with the Stars*.)

• • • • • • • •

Start: Place your right foot on the bench and your left foot on the floor.

Motion: Pushing through your right foot, straighten your right leg, drive up over the bench into a jump, and, in one motion, place your left foot down on the bench as you move your right foot off the bench and land it on the floor on the other side. Now repeat, driving up on your left foot. As you elevate over the bench, note your jump height. (You can do this by touching something overhead or just by paying attention to how high you're going.) Keep your pace undiminished over time; don't slow down and turn this into a pure strength exercise. If it's too easy and you never get tired, use a higher bench; otherwise it becomes a waste of time—a mere aerobic exercise, like step aerobics.

To minimize the risk of tripping or missing the bench as you get tired, start with a bench height of 12 inches.

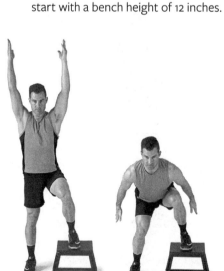
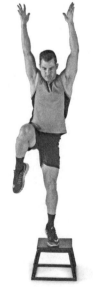
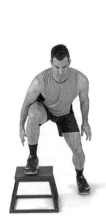

Classic Box Jump with a Step-Down

Why: A great power exercise

What it works: Quads, glutes, core, and coordination

· · · · · · · ·

Start: Stand with your feet at shoulder-width apart and a few inches away from and facing the box.

Motion: Lower into a squat and blast up, simultaneously throwing your hands back and then overhead. Lift your knees into your chest and straighten your legs as you land on the box. Step down one foot at a time to reduce the ballistic shock of the descent jump down.

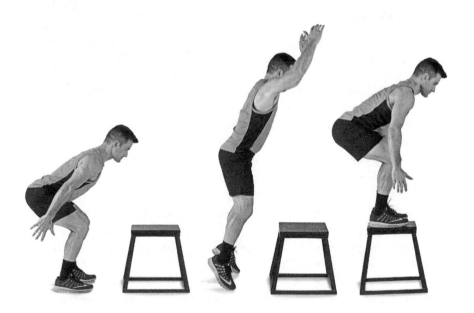

AT THE RACES

In his own words, here's what happened when one of a trio of Cat 2 and Cat 3 racers ranging in age from their 30s to their 50s trained with Maximum Overload.

TOD SMITH

"A 10 percent increase in wattage"

Age: 52

Occupation: Partner in a large accounting firm

Residence: Scottsdale, Arizona, and West LA

Level: Category 2 road racer

Accomplishment: 4th overall at the 2015 Tour of Scottsdale out of 50-plus riders, and "holding my own" in the 40-plus A race at Arizona's Tour of Gila 5-day stage race

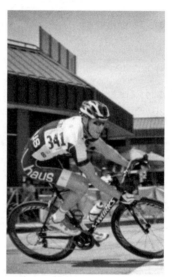

I have a long athletic résumé. I played sports growing up and started bike racing in 1982–83, back when LeMond was the man. I did it for many years, got into a few bad accidents. I got away from it when the kids were growing up, got back in heavily in my early 40s, and have been steady for the last decade.

I'm a good athlete, but not national championship level. I don't have a VO$_2$ max of 85, so I have to work very hard at it. And I do. I'm very focused on my nutrition and training—and pretty happy with the advice I got out of Jacques.

Maximum Overload was a fundamental change for me. I followed a traditional model, lifting weights in the off-season. But I needed to rebuild my muscle mass, which was declining with age.

I was riding well and very competitively on the local level, but I was having a hard time getting an incremental lift in my power; I felt there was something missing.

Someone told me I ought to talk to Jacques. I tracked him down; we had a couple meetings. That led to workouts beginning in 2012.

Although I had lifted, I did not understand the importance of strength to muscular endurance and explosiveness.

I stared seeing substantial benefit in 2 or 3 months. It took a while to build up but I saw good results. For a masters/aging athlete, I realized that training like a 24-year-old Italian doing stage races does not work. Jacques had me lifting throughout the year. It transformed my ability and my riding.

I actually got a 10 percent increase in wattage!

I've had more success on the local level since the Maximum Overload training. I have done comparative events like the Tour de Gila full 5-day stage race—holding my own in the 40-plus A race against Cat 1s, 2s, and 3s. I'm a Cat 2. I wasn't the only 50-plus rider, but I held my own.

I've had some top-10 stage results and have won a lot of races in Arizona. I got two podiums in five races in the 50-plus. In my last race, the Tour of Scottsdale last fall (2016), I was 4th overall out of 500-plus. One of the guys in front of me rides for BMC and did the Giro d'Italia.

I couldn't have done that without Jacques' training.

When I'm in LA, I'll go in and do a session with him. At home, I generally lift on Mondays and Thursdays. Before Jacques, I was lifting on my own only during the off-season, on Mondays.

Some small things regarding form and strategy have made a big difference for me. For instance, in doing the hex-bar deadlifts, he would have me set the weight down (unload the weight) each rep. That was a big change that transformed my ability. I also did a lot more one-leg presses. Did box jumps. More explosive stuff.

Jacques also transformed my body composition with my diet. I went away from eating sugar to a lot more healthy fat.

I'm busy, but I make the time to do the Maximum Overload workouts. They don't take long, but they pay off.

3

SELF-ASSESSMENT TESTS

We're all loaded with muscle imbalances, weak links, and biomechanical/postural limitations like kyphosis. Here's how to fix them so they don't hurt your Maximum Overload training—or hurt you.

When John Howard and Denise Mueller walked into the Sirens and Titans Fitness gym in West LA in January 2016, answered a Q&A, and did a few exercises, it didn't take Jacques DeVore long to see that he was going to have to write two different workout programs.

"Right now, Denise can deadlift heavy weight," he said. "But John can't—because he'll get injured.

"She can jump right into the program and move quickly from one exercise to another. His progress will be slower. His body is bent in the wrong places. On the walking lunge, he can't keep his hips down. On the deadlift, he can't bring his scapulas [shoulder blades] together. To do the exercises correctly and safely with heavy weights, he'll have to do extra drills first to straighten his body out.

"But once we get past that point, he'll take a big leap."

The subject of this chapter is the first step of the Maximum Overload plan: the all-important assessment. The assessment lets you know what kind of condition your body is in, how fast or slow you can jump into the program, and what extra drills you may need to safely prepare your body for the rigors of heavy weight training.

The assessment won't take long, and the drills work relatively fast to get you temporarily straightened out. But they absolutely cannot be skipped. The assessment and drills are so essential to the success of the Maximum Overload program that we have given them their own chapter—and we warn, plead, and beg you and everyone to use them.

And while this technically is a do-it-yourself assessment, we encourage you to do it along with someone who has some knowledge and background in weight training. After all, it can be difficult to see and evaluate your own movements.

Keep in mind that Denise Mueller is actually an anomaly in terms of weight-room familiarity. Far more cyclists, at every age and level of fitness, resemble Howard than her.

If you sit most of the day at a desk on a computer (like 99 percent of us) and are over 35, you most likely have some degree of kyphosis—a posture characterized by rounded-forward slump of the shoulders and upper back, a convex (not concave) lower back, and sucked-in glutes and hips. At the extreme, a kyphotic body posture is shaped like a corrupted C—not surprisingly, the same shape you take on when you sit at a desk or on a bike. Unless you actively do regular stretching/yoga and strength training (which most cyclists simply do not do—heck, that would cut into their riding time!), you most likely have a kyphotic posture. Kyphosis can be fixed, but not always easily; after years and years of relentless sitting and riding, your skeleton actually deforms.

Mueller, then 43 and being trained by Howard for an extreme bicycle-speed record attempt later that year, was not kyphotic. Quite robust, with great posture and thoracic spine mobility and stability, she had shoulders, hips, knees, and ankles that stacked up perfectly on a vertical line, humanity's standard factory setting. Her chest was proudly out, her shoulders and butt were proudly back, and her lower back was arched just right. In that configuration, standing tall and balanced against gravity, everything works perfectly. With muscles and joints all at the correct angles, there are no odd shearing forces on them that hinder efficiency, add stress, or lead to injury.

On top of that, Mueller loved going to the gym and had some experience lifting weights.

By contrast, Howard, the legendary three-time Olympian and Cycling Hall of Famer, was 68 and had severe kyphosis. His posture had the telltale C shape. He did no weight training and little stretching. And he did not own a gym membership.

Before DeVore considered letting Howard lift much weight—or even light weights—he had to try to de-slump his body, get more mobility in his upper spine, retract his scapulas, and get more hip mobility. "That lack of mobility forces his lower back to take more of the load than it is meant to," he explained. "Higher weights and volume would be risky for him."

That's why DeVore initially had Howard spend almost half of his Maximum Overload workout time on special drills and exercises that allowed his shoulder to be more mobile and added greater mobility to his upper spine, which pulled back his rounded shoulders and narrowed his spread-out shoulder blades. The result can be seen in the before-and-after photo on this page:

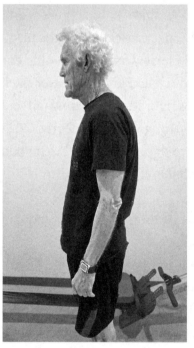 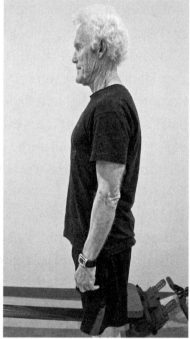

With his chest out, head up, and butt back after 20 minutes of drills, Howard lessened the severity of his slump, looked better, and actually gained an inch in height. Only then, properly straightened out, was he able to start lifting heavy weights *safely*, which stimulated the muscles to get stronger, more powerful, and fatigue resistant. (See the "fix-it" exercises below that Howard used.)

To summarize: When you are building something, whether it be a building, a car, or a body, you have to start with a sound foundation. You don't want to build a Ferrari on a bent frame. DeVore prefers to use an analogy from the arts: A body in perfect motion operates like an orchestra or a dance troupe. Stability, mobility, strength, power, and Maximum Sustainable Power (MSP) all come together in a symphony of *proprioceptive movement,* a rhythmic energy that flows as smooth as water. Your brain is the conductor, calling in the flutes, horns, and cymbals at exactly the right time, each instrument/body part aware of where it is in relation to the others. In the evaluation, we are looking for discordant notes, instruments that are out of tune—and fixing them. Otherwise the sound is terrible. If you don't fix them, you'll go slower on the bike and won't be able to lift the heavy weights at the gym that will improve you—and you might get injured trying.

Also, don't forget that an out-of-tune body affects you in normal life, too—with the prospect of back pain, aching joints, and chronic long-term health issues that magnify as you get older. If you're not careful, you can suffer a cascading effect, with an injury in one area leading to more injuries through the kinetic chain, say from hip to spine to upper back.

So Maximum Overload won't just make you a better cyclist. It'll make you healthier in real life. Along with MSP, you'll get better quality of life and increased longevity.

SELF-EVALUATION TESTS AND FIXES

On Day 1, grab a legal pad and a pencil and do a self-evaluation, the necessary first step in the Maximum Overload program (or any physical training, for that matter). Don't skip it, because it's your initial checkup, your opportunity to gauge your fitness level objectively (probably for the first time) and to see if all systems are go.

Naturally, everyone wants to jump immediately into the glamour exercises, the deadlift and the explosive walking lunge. But your ability to do those two and other heavily weighted exercises will be severely compromised and possibly lead to injuries if you don't do the self-examination first—and do it properly, then straighten your body out with special therapeutic exercises of mobility and stability if necessary.

Know this: You will find problems. No one is perfect. There will always be something, especially as you get older. Also, this will be an ongoing self-improvement program. As you improve shoulder mobility, you may find other weak links. As hip mobility increases, you'll need to improve spine mobility. Little by little, you'll check off all the weak links, yet always remain on guard for the new problems that inevitably crop up.

To begin the Maximum Overload exercises safely, you need to be able to perform basic movements properly and have adequate mobility and control of your body. Just a few minutes of drills can often temporarily correct posture and mobility problems enough to proceed with a modified version of the day's Maximum Overload workout. Over time, as you regularly do the mobility drills, your hips, lower back, and thoracic spine (T-spine) will open up and become more mobile, slowly turning back the clock as your body gets closer to its natural uncorrupted state.

Fully functional movement requires three things: **mobility** (the ability to move in a wide range of motion in your hips, shoulders, upper spine/T-spine, lumber/lower back, knees, ankles); **stability** (the ability to stay in place momentarily under control); and some minimal **strength.** Without the three, you get dysfunctional muscle activation—kind of a noodle-y feel—when doing most multijoint exercises.

Ready to do this? Sharpen your pencil and let's go!

Before the Test: Be Honest about Your Athletic History

As he did with Howard and Mueller, DeVore asks every client about his/her sports history. Those with no athletic background as a child or an adult must start the program slowly, as they have no muscle memory to tap. Everything for them will be new and strange. It's a different story for nonexercisers who haven't worked out in many years, yet played sports when young. They often can ramp up quick due to their muscle memory but still need to be patient with their progress.

Knowing your background not only sets up proper expectations, but also lets you understand your strengths and weaknesses. Sprinters have more explosive muscle development than long-distance cyclists and runners—you can tell by how high they can skip. They can get into the power exercises quicker. Mueller had ridden as a junior and stopped for 20 years, yet went to the gym several times a week. So she could jump into the program right away.

Note injuries. If you favor a bad hip, you will need to get it more mobile to lift heavy weights safely and/or lift lighter.

Step 1: Do the Overhead Squat Test

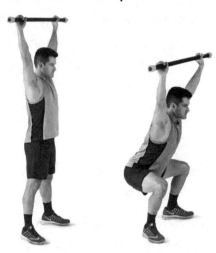

If you could do only one evaluation exercise, it would be the overhead squat. It gives you more information about total movement than anything else. It's simple: Try to hold a squat with a bar, broomstick, or towel overhead for 20 seconds, two or three times. This'll show you if your shoulders are mobile or immobile.

Squatting imperfections will indicate whether you have to slow down and work on technique and body-weight strength. Can you push your butt back and below the knees while keeping your head and shoulders up (as pictured in Chapter 2)? Are your hip flexors so tight that you can't get into a squat without your whole torso and shoulders being pulled excessively forward—and sit up straight, flatten your back, and pull the shoulders back? If you have poor T-spine mobility and tight shoulders, the weight of the bar will pull your arms down—you can't keep the bar vertical.

Also, do a low body-weight squat without the bar and observe the lower body. How low you can go, and are you leaning to one side or the other? This may indicate you may have hip, ankle, and knee mobility issues.

Step 2: Do the Dynamic Warm-Up Test

Don't be embarrassed if you struggle with the dynamic warm-up (see page 56). For some people, the dynamic warm-up *is* the workout. Some will quickly master the movements in a few rounds, while most will discover some mobility issues. If you can't do a body-weight walking lunge and keep your hips down and torso and head up, it may indicate shoulder, T-spine, and hip mobility issues.

Step 3: Do the Stability and Core Tests

If you can do the following basic movements without too much trouble, you have enough stability to begin lifting heavier weights. A good check: A month after you've started the program, do these tests again. It's a good way to see how much you've improved. No matter how good you were initially, you'll probably find that they'll be much easier than they were before.

These tests give feedback on how your body moves in everything you do. You may even find that after doing the program a while, it's easier to get out of bed or out of your car.

The exercises can be done in any order, as long you're warmed up.

Plank

This exercise relies upon anterior core (trunk) stability to keep you as stiff and straight as a board while suspended above the floor in a push-up position on your toes and elbows/forearms. Hold the plank for 1 minute. If you can't do it for 60 seconds, your trunk stability is weak. Work up to it with a knee plank.

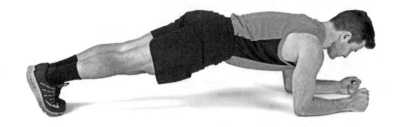

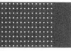

Shoulder Touch from Push-Up Position

From a push-up position, touch your right shoulder with your left hand; this checks rotational stability, which is key on a bike. After all, when you take your hand off the handlebar, you don't want to collapse. Also, rotational stability is important in a sprint for transferring power from your legs to your hands. Do 10.

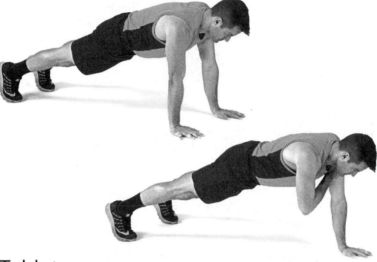

Tabletop

This exercise checks the strength of your lower back, which is important in climbing and on long-duration rides given that your power technically moves from your quads and glutes to your lower back. Anyone who has done a century or double-century knows how lower-back pain can slow you down. Start the tabletop on all fours with a flat back, and simply reach out and lift with your opposite arm and opposite leg in a quadruped position, then do the other side. Do 10.

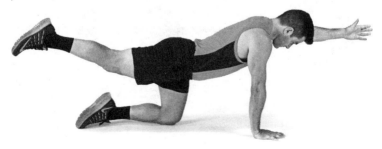

Suitcase Carry/ Farmer's Walk

This exercise works the core, upper body, and lower body and demonstrates their ability to work synergistically. Walk 10 steps with a dumbbell in each hand (20 pounds for men and 15 pounds for women), then come back. If you feel the weight is too light, add to the weight—you want the weight to feel heavy; In fact, some of you may ultimately carry as much as your full body weight between the two dumbbells. (Body builders will do long farmers walks to fire the little intercostal muscles.) Can you do six or seven steps without too much difficulty, no acute pain, and good posture and control? If so, your ability to tie upper and lower body together with your core is in pretty good shape.

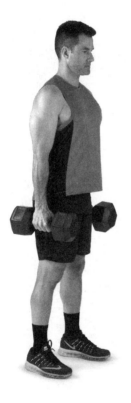
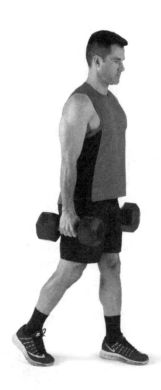

Waiter's Walk

This exercise demonstrates your shoulder stability, which is key on long rides, as you end up putting more weight on your upper body as the ride goes on (which is why the triceps often get fatigued on long days). Walk 10 steps with 15-pound (men) and 10-pound (women) dumbbells overhead and return. Make sure you can stabilize your shoulders without the weights waving around uncontrollably.

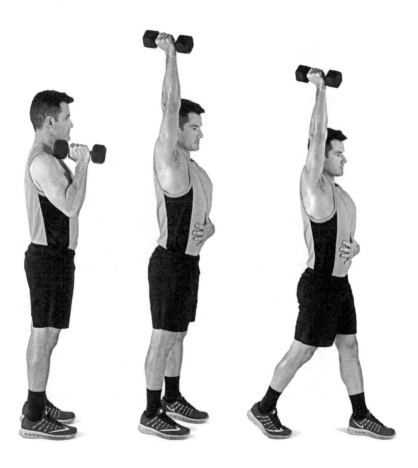

One-Leg Stand

This exercise identifies knee stability issues important in cycling. Stand on one leg and descend a couple inches by bending at the knee while holding your other leg out in front of your body. If you can do the movement and hold stability in the lowered position without knee pain or wobbliness, you're good to go.

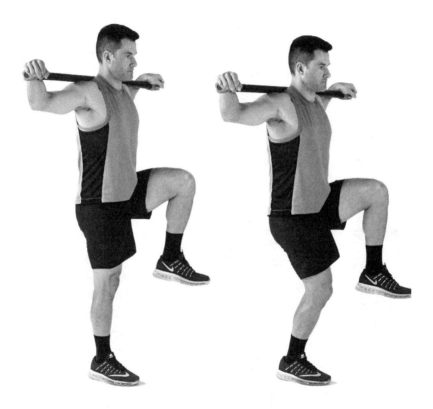

Reverse Lunge with Overhead Press

This exercise coordinates your upper and lower body, which work together in all cycling actions—sprinting, climbing, changing from a seated to standing position while ascending a hill. Use light weights: 5- to 15-pound dumbbells. Starting with both feet together and the weights held at your shoulders, step back into a lunge and simultaneously press the weight overhead. Try to hold that position steady for 5 to 10 seconds. If you have a harder time on one side or the other, you will identify weaknesses that you need to work on.

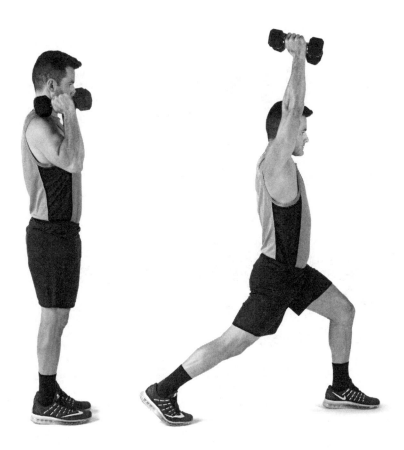

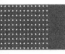

Trunk Stability Push-Up

This exercise can expose a glaring weakness for a cyclist. Do a normal push-up with hands at shoulder width and 6 to 8 inches forward of your head in a semi-Superman position. Inability to push up easily into this position indicates poor trunk stability. If you can't do it at all, pull your hands back inch by inch until you can do it.

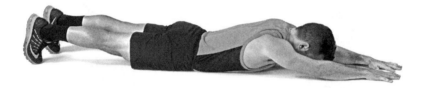

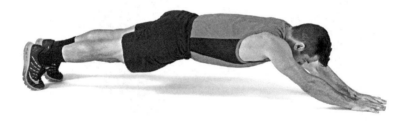

Overhead Ball Chop

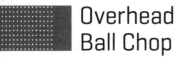

Start with a medicine ball over your head, and then lower your hips into a semi-squat as you swing it down between your legs. On the return trip back up, put it over the left shoulder instead of straight overhead. Swing down, and then return the ball up over your right shoulder. Alternate your movement between the left and the right. If you can't lower into the semi-squat, you need to work on hip mobility.

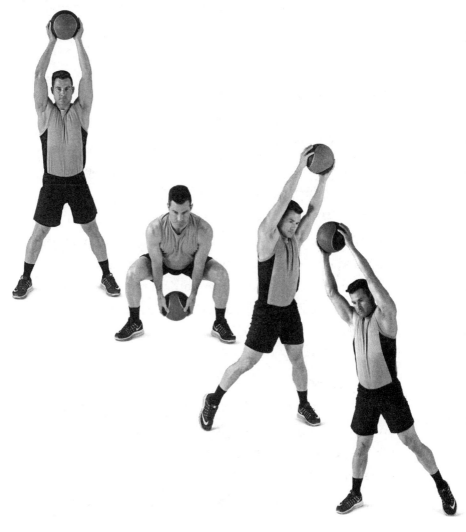

Step 4: Do Basic Strength Tests

These tests check for gross imbalances and weaknesses in the legs, lower body, and core. There must be enough equal-strength equivalency in the legs to do basic lower-body lifts safely. The upper body doesn't require as much strength—just enough to be able to hold a weighted bar. The core (including being able to do planks, addressed in Step 3 above) must be strong enough to support the kinetic chain and protect your back. Do not move on to heavy-weighted exercises until you can pass the basic strength tests below.

LOWER-BODY STRENGTH

a. Unweighted walking lunges, 10 reps

b. One-leg descents to a medium-height bench, 10 reps

c. Seated one-leg pistol squats, 10 reps. From a seated position on a bench, push yourself up, with your hands out in front as a counterbalance.

d. Seated squat. This is a test of hip strength in which you stand up out of a chair without the "old man getup"—hands on knees, leaning forward on the edge of the chair. Only 1 "rep" is required. Can you do it easily without using your arms to help?

UPPER-BODY STRENGTH

Note: Women typically have weaker upper bodies than men and often can't do many of these exercises initially. Don't worry; just keep trying. Gaining strength in these areas is essential to overall improvement.

a. Push-ups, 10 to 15 reps (men), 5 to 10 reps (women)

b. Dumbbell rows, 5 to 10 reps (men use 20 to 30 pounds; women use 15 to 20 pounds)

c. Dumbbell presses, 5 to 10 reps

d. Pull-ups, 3 reps (men), 1 rep (women)

These tests all help you to establish your baseline starting point.

CORE STRENGTH

a. AbDolly rollouts/body saw towel or ball slides, 5 to 10 reps

b. Reverse hyperextension on the ball, 5 to 10 reps

Note: The core, a key link in the kinetic chain from handlebars to pedals, is more than the abs; it's also the glutes, lower back, and everything between the hands and feet.

Step 5: Do the Absolute Power Output Jump Test

We use a jump here instead of lifting a weight because this is a power test, which by definition involves speed. Jumping is a good tool to measure if you are improving and can be done by height or length. We'll use the standing broad jump, which is safe and easy to measure.

Standing Broad Jump

You probably did this test in elementary school: From a standing position, squat, throw your arms back, and fly forward. To test your maximum power output, do three sets of 3 to 6 reps to failure, ending each set when you are too fatigued to maintain the distance. File your numbers away to be compared to a future test.

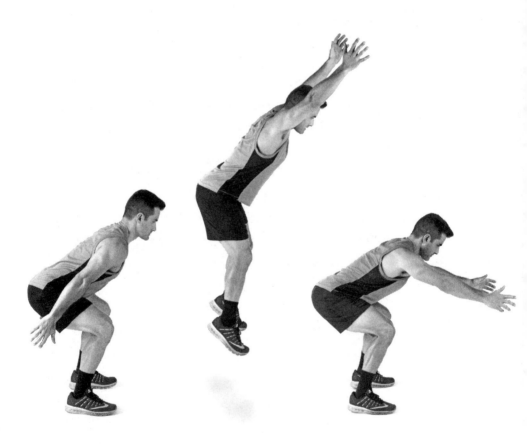

FIXING JOHN HOWARD (AND YOU) WITH TARGETED MOBILITY/CORRECTIVE EXERCISES

John Howard in many ways is a representative role model for all of us. An awesome aging athlete (who can still do things on a bike in his late 60s that most can't do at 20 or 30), he's been so focused on cycling throughout his life that he effectively gave up the ability to do other things, according to DeVore. He had significant but typical biomechanical issues with his shoulders, back, and hips—kyphosis, hip flexor tightness, and a weak upper body and could not touch his hands behind his back. That immobility and weakness delayed his Maximum Overload training with heavier weight exercises, which would have put his upper and lower back at risk and limited his ability to produce force.

A key rule of thumb in any training is this: Don't hurt yourself. "As a coach, my number-one job is not to injure the athlete," DeVore says. The fixes he recommended for Howard are appropriate for all of us, starting with an extended dynamic warm-up that includes several previously mentioned exercises—planks, shoulder-touch push-ups, and slow one-leg pistol squats—that activate the core and glutes, strengthen/reposition the torso, aid in mobility/stability in hips and T-spine, and allow the body to stabilize.

T-Spine and Shoulder Mobility Issues

According to DeVore, Howard was a "1 on a scale of 10—all caved over." He couldn't pull back his shoulders, retract his scapulas, or touch his hands behind his back, and he had a "turtle neck"—kyphotic shoulders that poked his neck forward.

Within minutes, the following T-spine mobility exercises loosened him up and straightened him out to the point where he looked noticeably better, stood taller, and was able to begin lifting heavier weights safely.

Bench Bar

This is a key exercise for people with restricted shoulder mobility. Kneel in front of a bench and place your arms on it, palms up, with your elbows centered in the middle of the bench. Using a bar or a single dumbbell, sit back on your heels, bring the bar/dumbbell overhead, and lower the weight behind your neck. Place it on your shoulders, forcing your chest down.

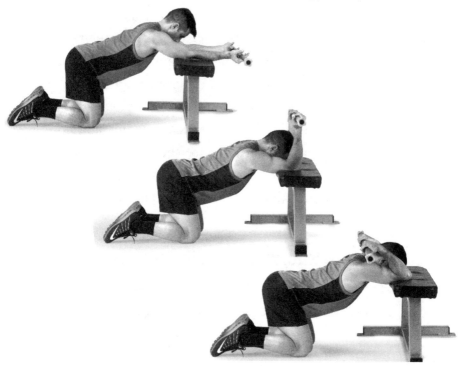

Foam Roller T-Spine Overhead Reach

This stretch helps restore a tall, concave shape to a rounded-forward back and shoulders by training you to retract your scapulas and open your chest. Lie on your back with your spinal column on a foam roller with your head and butt supported. Start with your hands stretched out vertically over your head, then slowly bring them down with the back of the hands toward the floor in the 90-degree crucifix ("Jesus") position. Raise and lower your arms to add to the stretch.

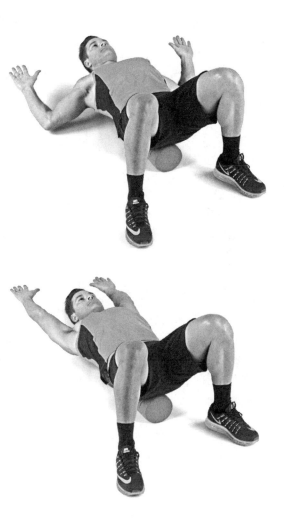

Overhead Band Pulses

To help open up slumped-forward shoulders, tie an elastic band to a pole at shoulder height and hold the untied end in one hand with your arm straight overhead. Step forward slightly so that there is a slight rear-pulling tension that pulls your arm back 5 to 10 degrees. Keeping your arm straight, pulse it forward vertically, then back, and repeat.

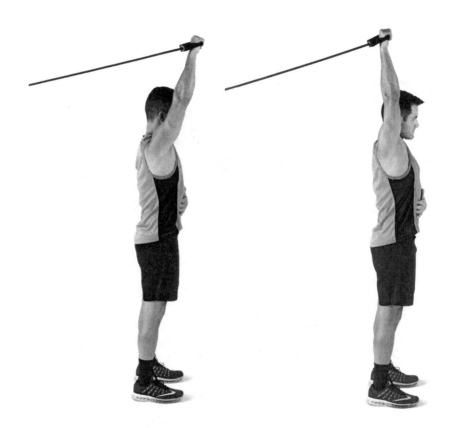

Rear Delt Band Exercise

This exercise fights the cyclists' hunched-over position by strengthening the rear deltoids and upper back. Gripping the ends of a stretch band in each hand with arms straight in front of you, pull your arms into a crucifix position and squeeze through your rear delts (i.e., go from the "Frankenstein" to the "Jesus" position).

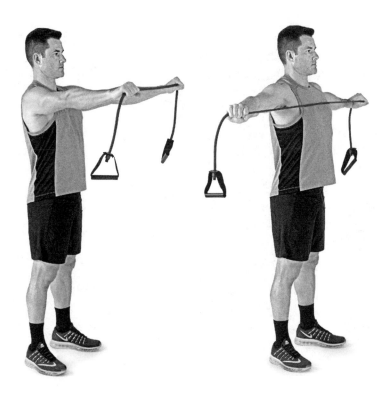

Cable Cross
High-Pull

This exercise also fights the cyclists' hunch, but uses a weight machine. Reach above your head and cross your arms in an X shape. Grab the handles and pull diagonally to the outside of the body with arms straight, ending with the hands/arms parallel.

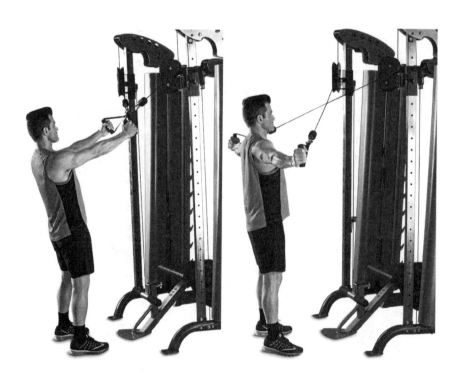

Hip Mobility

Tight, shortened hip flexors are an issue for nearly everyone in society, but especially cyclists. Lifelong racers like John Howard are at particular risk. In a seated position all day— on the bike, at the desk, in the car—he's always in a state of hip flexion, never extension. Use the following exercises to stretch out the hip flexors and restore natural flexibility, function and posture.

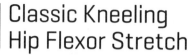

Classic Kneeling Hip Flexor Stretch

Kneel with one knee up and the other down on the floor behind you. While keeping a 90-degree angle at both knees and hips and your chest tall and vertical, squeeze your glutes, and focus on driving your hip forward and pressing the rear knee into the ground. This stretches the iliopsoas muscle, one of the main hip flexors.

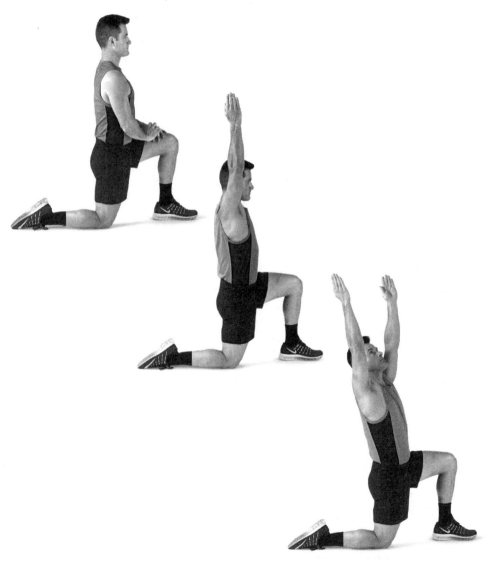

Foam Roll the Hip Flexors

Lying facedown across a foam roller, medicine ball, or lacrosse ball, apply pressure and drive it into the crease of your hip. Roll back and forth over tight, tender areas to maximize flexibility.

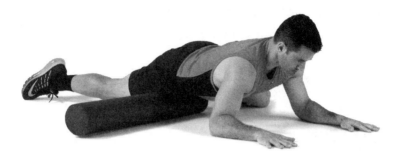

Couch Stretch

Originally performed against the arm of a couch (hence the odd name), this quad and hip flexor stretch starts by having you place your bent knee in the corner of a wall and the floor. Balancing on your opposite foot, push your erect back toward the wall. Until your flexibility increases, you may need to balance against a chair.

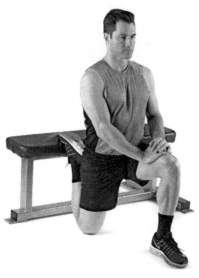

Knee Mobility

Like most cyclists, Howard has tight quads, which in some cases can cause lateral tracking of the kneecap. Note that cyclists generally don't have major knee issues, as cycling is forgiving to the knee (which is why the sport is crowded with former runners). A quick fix for both tight quads and tight hamstrings is as old school as you can get.

Side Lying Quad Stretch

There are various exercises to stretch your quad, but a safe, relaxing one is this: Lie on your left side with your head propped up, reach back with your right hand and pull your right foot toward your butt. Hold for 30 seconds, then switch sides.

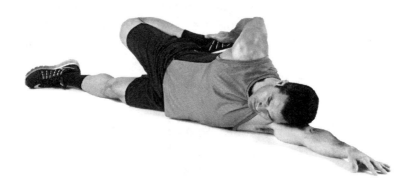

4

WHERE THE MAGIC HAPPENS: THE MAXIMUM OVERLOAD WORKOUT

Here's the safe, motivating, step-by-step sequence that builds to a dramatic grand finale challenge and creates Maximum Sustainable Power (MSP).

All the words you've read and the pictures you've seen in this book to this point are meaningless unless you get off your bike, head to the gym, and do the single thing in these pages that matters most: the workout.

The Maximum Overload workout will take you 40 to 60 minutes if you don't waste time. As you get fitter, it goes faster. It's set up as a progression that starts with dynamic warm-up body-weight movements; moves to core, back, and heavy-weight leg-strengthening exercises; then finishes with a special routine that addresses the underlying goal of the Maximum Overload program: raising your Maximum Sustainable Power (MSP)—i.e., your staying power on the bike, your ability to ride stronger longer. As you know by now, this MSP routine is conducted with explosive weighted walking lunges, an exercise that translates directly to cycling locomotion.

How hard, how heavy, and how fast do you make the MSP walking-lunge workout? Well, to force your body to make the greatest improvement in your MSP, the MSP walking-lunge workout by definition must be done at or as close as possible to your Absolute Power Output (APO). In practice, that means that you must do the lunges at as heavy as possible a weight that allows you to keep your speed. So you do not want to do them with very light weight at a superfast speed (because that simply becomes aerobic and isn't heavy enough to build power), or go so heavy that the weight slows you down, but at a weight and pace that are sustainably heavy and fast.

The concept is identical to your search for the right combination of gears and cadence on the bike. Remember the old high-school physics formula from Chapter 1: **Power = Strength x Speed**? Just as you would not use so big a gear on the bike that it bogs you down, you develop the greatest power from the MSP walking-lunge workout by finding a heavy weight that you can still move quickly. After all, what's the good of being stronger but slower?

USING APO TO FIND YOUR MSP

Since the weight of the dumbbells is so key to getting the MSP workouts right, how do you dial it in just right? Here, it is important to understand APO, which you've seen mentioned in the preceeding pages without a proper explanation. Basically, find your APO first, then use it to set up your MSP workout. That's because your goal with the MSP workouts, of course, is to spend a longer time at an increasingly high percentage of your APO.

What exactly is APO? Typically measured in watts, APO is an all-out, crazy-hard, short-term effort such as a sprint that you take to the point of "failure" (where you can't continue without slowing down or losing good form; see Chapter 6). A typical APO test on the bike might be a 30-second sprint. This gives you your baseline power. If your average power over this sprint is, say, 500 watts, your goal is to hold a high percentage of that number—say 350 watts—for longer and longer periods of time and eventually raise the number to 375 or 400 watts. By doing this, you've increased your MSP, the goal of the Maximum Overload program.

In the gym, DeVore has you take your APO test by doing 12 steps (that's 6 reps) of a walking lunge at a brisk velocity with a weight that doesn't slow you down, yet is so heavy that you reach failure (i.e., slow down or stop) by the 13th step. This is your baseline for the MSP workout, whose goal is to stretch out the time, number of steps, and overall cumulative overload at which you can carry those heavy dumbbells.

To stretch out your APO-established baseline, you rely on the secret sauce that makes Maximum Overload work: rest. Remember "the rest between the reps"? Using your APO-test dumbbell weights, break up the walking lunges into smaller sets of 5 or 6 steps and add rest in between.

For you formula freaks, the math is simple: **APO + Rest x Duration = MSP.**

Keep in mind that your APO will improve over time. You must retest every couple weeks to check the improvement. Keep upgrading the weights until they begin to bog down your speed and reduce your overall MSP totals.

DON'T SKIP STEPS. MSP IS THE GRAND FINALE

Before you get to the all-important MSP workout, remember that it is the last step, the grand finale of a deliberate sequence of preparatory exercises. Don't skip steps—you must do the exercises in order. For safety and effectiveness, DeVore found that you need to warm up the body methodically and activate the core and back muscles before hammering the prime mover muscles of the lower body with strength, then power, exercises. And psychologically, it has a very motivational flow, as the buildup gets you psyched for the big MSP workout at the end of the session.

The exercises used in the program, all detailed in Chapter 2, can be done in any gym with standard equipment: barbells, dumbbells, a leg-press machine, and a pull-up bar and/or lat-pull machine. Aside from the leg presses, you can do all the exercises at home with dumbbells and a pull-up bar.

Aside from using different weights, everyone follows the same Maximum Overload exercise lineup. Cyclists who have a weight-training background can usually begin lifting heavier weights right away, while the majority who have no lifting background start slower for safety and may have to do some of the additional mobility-enhancing, kyphosis-fighting exercises outlined in Chapter 3.

Generally, whether you start off weak or strong, most people will discover that their strength gains will begin to plateau after 4 to 6 weeks of twice-a-week workouts. Both experienced and inexperienced weight lifters alike will be surprised at how quickly they progress by lifting regularly.

THREE-PHASE STRENGTH-TO-POWER TIMELINE

Over the months, the Maximum Overload workout mix of exercises stays constant, but the emphasis changes as you progress through three phases: strength, APO, and your ultimate goal, MSP.

As you get into the nuts and bolts of each phase, remember that you can only build power on a foundation of strength, and that power is the result of adding velocity to strength. Strength toughens you up to withstand the MSP workouts. With that in mind, our first objective is to build strength by using heavy weight exercises like the deadlift.

The strength workouts get shorter, faster, and more time-efficient as you move into the power phases; this is because you can get by with abbreviated "maintenance"-strength exercise volume and sets (even though your strength still might improve a bit). You develop more power in the strong cycling-specific mover muscles by pushing moderately heavy weights as fast and as long as you can with a dynamic exercise like the explosive walking lunge. It's essential that you do a regular biweekly APO test with the walking lunge to gauge your rise in absolute power, but stop adding weight when you find that it slows you down.

Day 1: Do the Assessment

If you can pass the overhead squat test, the dynamic warm-up test, the stability and core test, and all the basic strength tests noted in Chapter 3, it means that you have enough mobility in your knees, hips, and shoulders to jump right into Phase 1, Maximum Overload's strength-building workouts. Otherwise, keep doing the aforementioned until your body is ready.

Phase 1—Weeks 1 to 4: Build Strength

If you don't build strength before you build power, you won't have a foundation that can support and withstand the rigors of fast, powerful movements. So you do multijoint movements to overload for 3 to 4 weeks to strengthen everything: the upper body, the lower body, and the core. Now, an old analogy again applies: Building strength is like putting better

HOW TO FIND YOUR STARTER WEIGHTS FOR STRENGTH EXERCISES

Remember, strength exercises like the deadlift are "grunting" exercises. The weight will be heavy, so the movement will be slow. Speed is not part of the equation, as it is with power exercises like the walking lunge

With the deadlift, the goal is to find the maximum weight you can pick up off the floor for 6 to 8 reps. To find your starter baseline weight, initially do 10 deadlifts with a 10-pound dumbbell in each hand, then ask yourself: "Was the tenth rep a struggle?" For 99 percent of you, it shouldn't be, so repeat with 15-pound dumbbells. If you maintain form and pace for 8 to 10 reps, go to 20 pounds, then to an unweighted 45-pound bar. Once you can't do 8 to 10 reps without a struggle, you've found the starter weight with which to officially begin the workouts. After that, never raise the weight over 10 percent from one session to the next.

Note: Always start the first set with a warm-up "indicator set"—a lighter weight and 12 reps. That'll probably be enough to indicate or reveal any strange aches or pains and let you know if all systems are "go."

tires on the car: Now you can safely test the speed—push it to 50, 60, 100 mph (i.e., ramp up power)—without blowing the tires (your ligaments, bones, connective tissue).

Strength will increase rapidly in the first 3 weeks (assuming two workouts per week). After that, progress slows and big jumps won't occur as rapidly anymore. You will establish your foundation when you begin to plateau.

Rules for "strength" exercises: You need a foundation of strength to build the ultimate goal of this program—power. So the goal of the back and lower-body strength exercises is to lift the heaviest possible weights, while keeping good form. Check the tutorials in Chapter 2; do not progress until your form is correct; otherwise you'll risk injury and compromise your performance.

Reps and sets: A tried-and-true strength-building protocol uses four sets of increasing weight with decreasing number of reps to near failure (the point at which it will be too difficult to do another rep correctly). The given rep ranges (Set 1: 10 reps; Set 2: 8 reps; Set 3: 6 reps; and Set 4: 3 reps) are ideal for building the strength you need as a foundation for subsequent power work. Set 1 is a warm-up set with light weights. Use the warm-up time to listen to your body; if you detect strange aches and pains, do more warm-up, reduce your weight increases, or stop altogether. Newbie lifters should do additional warm-up reps to dial in their form.

Weight: Set the weight heavy enough that you max out at the given rep count (meaning if 3 reps is the goal, you can't finish 4 or more reps). *Note:* DeVore does not prescribe 1-rep-max lifting. "There's not that much advantage for someone whose sport is not weight lifting," he says. "The risk-return is not that good."

Phase 2—Weeks 5 to 8: Build APO As You Keep Building Strength

Once you have strength, you add speed in order to raise your Absolute Power Output (APO). The mechanism for this is a sequence of power exercises, which includes the preferred explosive walking lunge as well as wall ball, thruster, box jumps, push press, kettlebells, and others mentioned in Chapter 2. You've already been doing some of these exercises during Phase 1. Now you focus on finding your maximum benchmark weight where you produce the greatest amount of power. You will test this over a 12-step set of walking lunges (note that 12 steps = 6 steps on each leg). All the while, you will still maintain and even incrementally improve your deadlift and other strength exercises but spend less time on them, doing a 12-rep warm-up and two or three 6-rep sets to maintain the strength that you developed in the previous strength phase.

Phase 3—Weeks 9 to 12: Build MSP

At the end of the second month, having found your maximum benchmark weight via the APO test, which serves as a baseline for your walking-lunge Maximum Sustainable Power (MSP) workout, you now lengthen your efforts. (You are not going to increase the APO too much from here, but you will increase how long you can sustain the highest percentage of this newfound APO.) You are going to extend the time periods of the workout, growing your MSP as you push the duration of the lunge sets from 1 minute to 2 minutes to 4 minutes in 15- or 30-second increments. Remember the correlation: The longer you can extend the time on the lunges, the longer you'll be able to hold a higher percentage of your APO on a hill climb or hard effort on the bike.

Reminder: Keep your velocity up. If your speed drops off more than 10 to 15 percent, stop the workout. Suboptimal workouts do not improve MSP. If you fly through 20-pound lunges, raise the weight to 25. But if 30 pounds bog you down, go back to 25.

THE MAXIMUM SUSTAINABLE POWER (MSP) WORKOUT

Do the exercises in order: As mentioned at the outset of this chapter, don't mess with the sequence of the exercises: warm-up, core, back strength, lower-body strength, lower-body power. For safety, psychology, and performance, the sequence prepares your body and mind for a rousing, session-ending MSP workout that will build your ability to hold watts longer. Get ready for the first time that you look at your power meter and say, "Holy crap, I was able to hold 300 watts so much longer than I did last time on that a climb." Raising your MSP is the whole point of the program.

Frequency and rest: Do the full Maximum Overload workout one to three times a week in the preseason and one time a week or every other week in season. Be careful at first; these workouts can be taxing. They will make you sore. If you jump into three workouts right away, you won't be able to walk. Besides getting you the necessary recovery time, rest helps you keep your velocity up on the next workout. Muscles must be fresh to work at maximum efforts.

Rules for "Power" Exercises

Remember that there are two goals here:

1. Establish your APO baseline with three sets of 10 reps. Then . . .

2. Increase the time of your MSP workout with the mini-sets.

Since power (Power = Strength x Speed) is the goal of all of this work, the workout always follows strength work with power exercises. To teach your muscles to produce the greatest amount of power, you must first develop your APO, then extend it over time to achieve your ultimate goal, MSP. DeVore says that your ultimate MSP goal should be at 75 to 85 percent of your APO. For example: If you reach your APO in the walking lunge with 45-pound dumbbells, your goal in the MSP workout would be to use 30- to 35-pounders in your three-lunge mini-sets.

Note: It's a good idea to do the first MSP set at a lower weight. That's what Denise Mueller would do to get her rhythm.

Again, beware of going too light and too slow. Going too light will let you speed through the routine for a long time, but that turns this into an endurance event, which isn't the goal. On the flip side, if speed drops off more than 10 or 15 percent, you are no longer producing a high enough power to add any benefit. This is what we call "submaximal effort," which gives you submaximal results. You must operate at near-absolute power output longer to push up your MSP.

Reps and sets: APO is developed in sets of 6 to 8 reps (in the walking lunge, 1 rep = 2 steps). Remember: Too many reps turns a set into an endurance exercise; once you get past 8 reps, your power output diminishes greatly and it becomes a suboptimal endurance effort. Rest is key. Start with a 10- to 15-second rest between mini-sets, and raise or lower as needed. If you drop below 85 percent of maximum power at any time, stop and rest.

It takes about 3 to 4 weeks to top off your APO. Using the recommended explosive walking lunges as per the workout schedule below, that means finding the heaviest dumbbells you can hold while keeping the highest velocity for 1 minute. In the sample schedule, you work up to and plateau at 35-pounders. Then, using the 35s, you gradually push your walking-lunge time up to a maximum of 4 minutes. This training scheme allows your body to adapt to long outputs at MSP. You will not produce any more APO, but you will be able to hold a much higher percentage of it.

This same principle works for intervals, which will be discussed in Chapter 6, and they are incorporated into the overall Maximum Overload weights/bike training schedule. The intervals length would be matched to the event or sport.

Here's a template of the Maximum Overload weight-lifting plan:

I. Dynamic Warm-Up

Do two sets of 12 reps of each:

1. Walking Lunge with spine-mobility twist (page 59)
2. Sidestep Hip Mobility Lunge with Arms Up (page 60)
3. Stretch-Band Lateral Side Shuffle (page 61)
4. Cowboy Walk with bands (page 62)
5. Hip-Thrust/Glute Bridge (page 63)
6. High-Knee Skip (page 64)

II. Core Strength

Do three sets of 12 reps of two of these exercises (mix and match as you prefer):

1. Reverse Hyper on physio ball (page 66)

2. Static Plank and Pelvic-Tilt Plank (page 67)

3. AbDolly Rollout and Body Saw with towel/physio ball (page 68)

III. Back Strength

1. Bent-Over Dumbbell Row (page 70). Do three sets of increasing weight to your max at 10 reps, 6 reps, and 3 reps.

2. Close-grip Lat Pulldown (page 72) or Pull-Up (page 71). For the lat pulls, do three sets of increasing weight to your max at 10, 6, and 3 reps, focusing on retracting the scapulas into the center of your back. For pull-ups, try to do your max each time.

IV. Lower-Body Strength

1. Single-Leg Press (page 80). Warm up with 10 light-weight double-leg presses, then do single-leg presses: three sets of increasing weight to your max at 10, 6, and 3 reps. For example: Do 10 reps at 135 pounds, 6 reps to 180 pounds; 3 reps to a max of 200 pounds.

2. Hex/Trap Bar Deadlift (page 76). Do three sets of increasing weight to your max at 10, 6, and 3 reps. For

example: 10 reps at 140 pounds; 6 reps at 210 pounds; 3 reps at 230 pounds.

3. Romanian Deadlift (page 78). Do three sets of increasing weight to your max at 10, 6, and 3 reps. For example: 10 reps at 95 pounds; 6 reps at 115 pounds; 3 reps at 145 pounds.

4. Goblet Squat. This is a squat with a dumbbell held with both hands in front of your body. Do three sets of increasing weight to your max at 10, 6, and 3 reps. For example: 10 reps at 35 pounds; 6 reps at 45 pounds; 3 reps at 60 pounds.

5. "Deep" Push Press/Thruster (page 88). Do three sets of increasing weight to your max at 10, 6, and 3 reps.

Note: If you want to reduce the total exercise time, interlace the exercises with noncompeting exercises. For example: Follow a lower-body exercise with an upper-body exercise, like a pulldown. That'll still provide 3 to 4 minutes of rest for the legs. You can throw several exercises in the mix. If you started with hyperextensions, go to the AbDolly and pulldowns and finish with the hex/trap bar deadlift.

V. Lower-Body Power and the Maximum Sustainable Power (MSP) Workout

1. Warm up with Thrusters (page 88) or Wall Ball (page 90), three sets of 10 reps with light weights

2. Do the Maximum Sustainable Power (MSP) workout with forward-weighted Explosive Walking Lunges (page 86).

WEEK-BY-WEEK PROGRESSION OF THE MAXIMUM SUSTAINABLE POWER (MSP) WORKOUT USING THE EXPLOSIVE WALKING LUNGE

Your ultimate goal is taking as many steps as possible with as heavy a weight as possible, while still maintaining your speed. Keep adding sets and toying with the best combination of weight, rest, and steps.

Start with three sets of 1 minute each with a nominal amount of weight in each hand. As you get the form down, progress to heavier weights and a 2-minute set length through Week 4. Keep your form and pace perfect throughout.

From Weeks 5 to 8, build your MSP by keeping the sets at 2 minutes in duration while raising the weight as high as possible as you maintain your speed (step count) and form.

From Weeks 9 to 12, build your MSP by extending the set duration for the explosive walking lunge from 2 minutes to 4 minutes. For a sample progression see pages 142 to 148.

Closer to the season, as you get fitter, DeVore recommends that you settle on a weight, reduce the rest time, and focus on extending your workout time and overall MSP step count.

Note: Record keeping is essential for maintaining the effectiveness and motivation of the MSP workouts; the numbers let you know that you're improving. For each set, add up the total weight lifted. Keep your totals for each set and the each entire MSP workout. For example: If you did 40 steps with 30-pound dumbbells in each hand in a 2-minute set, your total is 2,400 pounds (40 steps x 60 pounds [30 pounds x 2 hands]). This is described in more detail in the next section.

Phase 1: Build Your Power Base under Load, Exercise Skill, and Duration to 2-Minute Sets

Week 1 Workout

Goal: Do a 1-minute MSP workout. Get comfortable with the movement. You may stay with 1-minute durations for a month if necessary, or skip to Weeks 3 and 4 and 2-minute durations. Everyone progresses differently based on his or her fitness and skills. The 20-pound baseline weight listed below is just a sample; you might feel more comfortable starting with a 10-pound weight.

Set 1: 20 lbs. in each hand. Do repeats of 6 steps + 10- to 15-sec. rest for 1 min.

Set 2: 20 lbs. (6 steps + 10- to 15-sec. rest) for 1 min.

Set 3: 20 lbs. (6 steps + 10- to 15-sec. rest) for 1 min.

Note:

- 6 steps = 3 steps on each leg.
- Don't go beyond a 15-second rest; the sets must be kept close enough to build MSP. If so, you may have to start at a lower weight—there's nothing wrong with that.
- If you feel that you can squeeze in 8 consecutive steps and still recover, then go for it. You are not wedded to

6 steps per mini-set. This applies to all workouts from this point. Also, you can shorten the rest time, but don't lengthen beyond 10 to 15 seconds. The goal is to maximize your overload of power for the entire workout during the allotted time frame.

Week 2 Workout

Goal: Extend MSP time to 1:30 without slowing the speed of your lunges.

Set 1:   20 lbs. (6 steps + 10- to 15-sec. rest) for 1 min.

Set 2:   20 lbs. (6 steps + 10- to 15-sec. rest) for 1:30

Set 3:   20 lbs. (6 steps + 10- to 15-sec. rest) for 1:30

Week 3 Workout

Goal: Extend MSP time to 2 minutes without slowing.

Set 1:   20 lbs. (6 steps + 10- to 15-sec. rest) for 1:30

Set 2:   20 lbs. (6 steps + 10- to 15-sec. rest) for 2:00

Set 3:   20 lbs. (6 steps + 10- to 15-sec. rest) for 2:00

Week 4 Workout

Goal: Raise your step count, keep speed and 2-minute duration.

Set 1:   20 lbs. (8 steps + 10- to 15-sec. rest) for 1:30

Set 2:   20 lbs. (8 steps + 10- to 15-sec. rest) for 2:00

Set 3:   20 lbs. (8 steps + 10- to 15-sec. rest) for 2:00

Phase 2: Keep the 2-Minute Duration, but Raise MSP and Total Overload by Adding More Weight

Week 5 Workout

Goal: Maintain your step count and raise your APO. These numbers assume that your new APO baseline is 25 pounds. As you get better at this, the weight will become too light, so test and raise it. On the second set, bump the weight up and drop the steps to 6.

Set 1: 20 lbs. (8 steps + 10- to 15-sec. rest) for 2:00

Set 2: 25 lbs. (6 steps + 10- to 15-sec. rest) for 2:00

Set 3: 25 lbs. (6 steps + 10- to 15-sec. rest) for 2:00

Week 6 Workout

Goal: Increase your step count to 8, which increases the overload from the week before. If you feel that your velocity is too high and the weight is too light, do an APO test to reset your 10-steps-to-failure baseline weight.

Set 1: 20 lbs. (8 steps + 10- to 15-sec. rest) for 2:00

Set 2: 25 lbs. (8 steps + 10- to 15-sec. rest) for 2:00

Set 3: 25 lbs. (8 steps + 10- to 15-sec. rest) for 2:00

Week 7 Workout

Goal: Maintain your step count and raise your APO baseline. Assume your new baseline is 30 pounds.

Set 1: 25 lbs. (8 steps + 10- to 15-sec. rest) for 2:00

Set 2: 30 lbs. (6 steps + 10- to 15-sec. rest) for 2:00

Set 3: 30 lbs. (6 steps + 10- to 15-sec. rest) for 2:00

Week 8 Workout

Goal: Raise your step count and raise your total overload. If you feel that your velocity is too high and the weight is too light, test to reset your 10-steps-to-failure APO baseline weight.

Set 1: 30 lbs. (8 steps + 10- to 15-sec. rest) for 2:00

Set 2: 35 lbs. (8 steps + 10- to 15-sec. rest) for 2:00

Set 3: 35 lbs. (8 steps + 10- to 15-sec. rest) for 2:00

Phase 3: Build Maximum Sustainable Power (MSP) and Raise Maximum Overload by Maintaining the Weight and Extending the Workout Duration to 3 or 4 Minutes

Week 9 Workout

Goal: Now at your maximum APO weight, raise your step count and your overload by extending time to 2:30.

Set 1: 30 lbs. (8 steps + 10- to 15-sec. rest) for 2:30

Set 2: 35 lbs. (6 steps + 10- to 15-sec. rest) for 2:30

Set 3: 35 lbs. (6 steps + 10- to 15-sec. rest) for 2:30

Week 10 Workout

Goal: Change your MSP overload by extending time to 3 minutes.

Set 1: 30 lbs. (8 steps + 10- to 15-sec. rest) for 3:00

Set 2: 35 lbs. (6 steps + 10- to 15-sec. rest) for 3:00

Set 3: 35 lbs. (6 steps + 10- to 15-sec. rest) for 3:00

(continued on page 148)

AT THE RACES

In his own words, here's what happened when one of a trio of Cat 2 and Cat 3 racers ranging in age from their 30s to their 50s trained with Maximum Overload.

BRAD WILLIAMS

"Maintained speed on less training"

Age: 35

Occupation: Architect

Residence: West Los Angeles

Level: Category 3 road racer for 3 years, triathlete/bike racer for 5

Accomplishment: Finished 20th in Cat 3s at the 2014 Brentwood Grand Prix, a big local race. Trained with DeVore 2 years at the time of this interview (spring 2016)

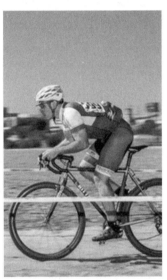

After working out with Jacques, you are strong. STRONG. You can really mash on the pedals. And you have confidence you can push on the pedals as well as anyone in the group.

Before this, I'd already been going to the gym to supplement my cycling. I was doing double-leg presses. I thought I was pretty badass because I could do a bunch of weight. I didn't understand that just being strong doesn't do a lot of good. Jacques told me, "First we're going to make you strong, then we're going to make you fast, then we are going to make you powerful."

It's almost like a pyramid. You have strength, and you have speed. And when you get both, you can build power. Then from that, you can build sustainable power.

And I did. I stayed as fast as I ever was while training half the time. At the peak of the previous racing season, where I was on my bike all the time, my peak threshold power was around 250 watts. Then we had a baby, and I was no longer able to ride two or three times during the week, only doing my long weekend ride. Yet I lost no speed at all.

With Jacques, I was able to re-create my old threshold power level on a fraction of the riding—perfect for a guy with a kid. I was riding less, yet I was able to maintain because I was as strong as an ox. My cardio fitness was not up to my standard, but I could continue to keep up in training and in races. It helped bridge a gap for me at the time. I was riding less for sure, couldn't do 3- to 4-hour rides every weekend. This was a much more efficient, focused 45-minute/1-hour workout.

If I was to speculate, the Maximum Overload workout is best at replacing two or three smaller rides during the week. Not a two- to three-hour ride, but it may take the place of focused intervals.

I met Jacques on a racing team, which soon shut down after that, then bumped into him at a bike shop where he was doing a class on maximum sustainable power. I came into his gym and started doing VersaClimber and lighter weight classes, then went to one-on-one training with him twice a week, building strength and building speed.

We do all the big strength exercises: hex-bar deadlifts, Romanian deadlifts, single-leg presses. And to build the fast muscle response, we do the speed exercises: VersaPulley short rows, the MVP machine. I do the maximum sustainable power test mainly on the VersaPulley, with some explosive walking lunges.

Once in a while when I'm out of town, I'll do some of the exercises on my own in a regular gym: box jumps, leg presses, and Romanian deadlifts with a straight bar. I have told my small circle of racers about my training, but it fell on deaf ears because they are very traditional and don't do weights.

I got hit by a car last year—it pulled out in front of me on October 25, 2015. I got five broken vertebrae. I'm still rehabbing. I can walk normally, I'm healed, but I'm still gaining strength. Once I got clearance from my surgeon, I jumped back in the weight room with Jacques.

I feel very lucky. Jacques picked up right where my physical therapist left off. They have approached my rehab identically. He's ramping it up. I'm aiming for my baseline before I got hurt.

Week 11 Workout

Goal: Raise your step count and raise your overload by extending time to 3:30.

Set 1:   30 lbs. (8 steps + 10- to 15-sec. rest) for 3:30

Set 2:   35 lbs. (6 steps + 10- to 15-sec. rest) for 3:30

Set 3:   35 lbs. (6 steps + 10- to 15-sec. rest) for 3:30

Week 12 Workout

Goal: Change your MSP overload by extending time to 4 minutes.

Set 1:   30 lbs. (8 steps + 10- to 15-sec. rest) for 4:00

Set 2:   35 lbs. (6 steps + 10- to 15-sec. rest) for 4:00

Set 3:   35 lbs. (6 steps + 10-sec. rest) for 4:00

5

THE BIG PICTURE: 3 MONTHS TO SUPER CYCLING

How the 12-week Maximum Overload training schedule fits into a comprehensive cycling training program

Now that Maximum Overload and its goal of Maximum Sustainable Power (MSP) have been explained in detail, let's look at the big picture: how this unique performance-enhancing weight-training program for endurance athletes fits within the broader context of a comprehensive daily/weekly cycling training program.

Jacques DeVore stresses that Maximum Overload works for every type of rider—competitive racers, century riders, enthusiasts, and not-so enthusiasts—and is complementary to traditional coaching and training plans. Sequenced correctly to allow for proper recovery, it works with intervals, tempo rides, hard group rides, and cross-training. He also believes that the results of the Maximum Overload training plan are improved by a natural-food diet light on processed carbs and sugars, which is healthier for you in the long run and encourages fat-burning and weight loss, key issues in a power-to-weight-ratio sport like cycling. The rest of the book is devoted to a discussion of these issues.

This chapter is short and simple, but important, as it shows how Maximum Overload workouts are embedded into a normal daily/weekly training schedule. It lays out weekly off-season and in-season training schedules for serious and recreational riders alike.

DeVore says that Maximum Overload can be started at any time of the year, because getting stronger and more powerful will help everyone of any ability, but that the off-season is obviously the best starting point. Serious riders, freed of worrying over keeping up with the competition in the off-season, have time in the fall and winter to experiment stress-free and get through the muscle discomfort and slowness of the first couple weeks, when the body is getting used to the new overload.

Two or three sessions of Maximum Overload per week in the off-season and once a week during the season can fit fairly easily into your existing training schedule. It fills in for existing rest days (usually Mondays for racers) and gives you purpose on dark winter and bad weather days. It's a big time-saver for several reasons: A 1-hour Maximum Overload workout can replace and improve upon a hard 3-hour training ride, says DeVore. It'll deepen your muscular power to the point where you get more overload out of each pedal stroke, thereby increasing the training effect on each training ride—so your rides can be shorter—and even slot into a traditional off day: Most competitive cyclists take Monday off, so why not go to the gym that night?

To make the workouts most effective and less disruptive of your normal riding, keep these rules in mind.

- **Try not to ride hard the day before a Maximum Overload (MO) workout.** Come to the gym fresh, so that you can do maximal efforts. Maximal efforts yield maximum results; submaximal yields submaximal results.

- **Don't ride hard the day after a MO workout.** Your legs will feel crummy, especially in the first month, as your body struggles to get used to pushing heavy weights. Don't freak out at how slow you are. Initially, the day after a MO workout, you will be slower. But like a fog, that will lift as your muscles strengthen and the trauma of the initial weight workouts dissipates.

- **Experienced gym-goers can ramp it up.** To accelerate strength gains, cyclists with some weight-lifting or CrossFit experience can schedule three MO workouts per week (Monday, Wednesday, Friday) for the first 2 or 3 weeks.

- **New to weights? Go light at first.** Weight-room newbies and those intimidated by heavier weights may find that a three-MO-a-week format with light weights may work for you. Use the lighter weights until you get comfortable. Once that happens, go to the standard twice-a-week schedule.

- **Lift less in season.** As the season progresses and riding time increases, MO drops to one session per week. Here's the progression: **You can ride less.** Once you develop newfound power in the gym, you can **ride less yet get fitter as you ride.** That's because you will not only go faster on the bike, but you will also get a better workout since all your rides will be at higher overloads.

Month 1: **2 or 3 MO workouts/week.** Goals: Build strength and establish absolute power output (APO) baselines.

Month 2: **2 MO workouts/week.** Goal: Continue to build power and strength (i.e., raise your APO). The second MO workout leaves out the walking-lunge MSP workout to spare your legs for weekend rides.

Month 3: **2 MO workouts/week.** Goal: Raise MSP. The second MO workout leaves out the walking-lunge MSP workout to spare your legs for weekend rides.

In season: **MO once a week.** Goals: Raise or maintain strength/MSP.

12-WEEK OFF-SEASON TRAINING OVERVIEW

STANDARD OFF-SEASON WEEK AT A GLANCE

Monday: MO workout

Tuesday: Easy ride

Wednesday: MO workout, but only do the APO test (not an MSP) on Week 4.

Thursday: Tempo ride or intervals

Friday: Active recovery ride

Saturday: Big long aerobic ride or optional MO workout

Sunday: Easy shorter ride

Weeks 1 to 4: Self-Evaluate and Build Strength

Goal: Get your body ready for the new stresses of weight lifting by identifying biomechanical/postural inefficiencies, learning the proper form of the exercises, and establishing some general strength baselines for your deadlifts and other exercises. You'll do an APO test in Weeks 1 and 4. And you'll do a 1-minute MSP. You are learning how to execute MSP effectively. Common sense dictates that you should not test yourself with heavy weights until you straighten out you body as much as possible with the warm-up, remedial, and core exercises and have a high confidence in your technique. Unless you're a CrossFitter or experienced gym rat, these exercises will be new to you, and you will hurt. That's okay—

CALENDAR 1 (WEEKS 1 TO 4):
SELF-EVALUATE AND BUILD STRENGTH

	SUNDAY	MONDAY	TUESDAY	
WEEK 1	Off day, cross-train, or easy short spin	Maximum Overload workout starting with 1-minute MSP	Easy long slow distance (LSD) ride	
WEEK 2	Off day, cross-train, or easy short spin	Maximum Overload workout, raising MSP to 1:30	Easy LSD ride	
WEEK 3	Off day, cross-train, or easy short spin	Maximum Overload workout, raising MSP to 1:45	Easy LSD ride	
WEEK 4	Off day, cross-train, or easy short spin	Maximum Overload workout, raising MSP to 2:00	Easy LSD ride	

you just don't want to get injured, which is easy to do in the early going by plunging in due to pure enthusiasm.

Although the schedule here calls for two Maximum Overload days per week, with a PAP option of adding intervals on Wednesday and a Saturday MO in lieu of a long ride, back off if you get too beat-up. Get active recovery with an easy ride or cross training the days after a MO workout to enhance blood-flow and reduce soreness.

Week 1

The primary objective in Week 1 is to self-evaluate your body and learn proper exercise form. Determine if you have to address biomechanical issues (we all have them). Establish

WEDNESDAY	THURSDAY	FRIDAY	SATURDAY
Maximum Overload workout. Optional: Follow with intervals.	Tempo/LSD ride or easy cross-training day	Active recovery ride	Alternative MO workout or big long aerobic ride
Maximum Overload workout. Optional: Follow with intervals.	Tempo/LSD ride or easy cross-training day	Active recovery ride	Alternative MO workout or big long aerobic ride
Maximum Overload workout. Optional: Follow with intervals.	Tempo/LSD ride or easy cross-training day	Active recovery ride	Alternative MO workout or big long aerobic ride
Maximum Overload workout. Optional: Follow with intervals.	Tempo/LSD ride or easy cross-training day	Active recovery ride	Alternative MO workout or big long aerobic ride

your baseline APO and strength baselines for all upper body, lower body, and core exercises, such as your 6-rep deadlift max. Then establish a baseline for your MSP workout. Can you hold your APO for 30 seconds—or 1 minute? (Remember: APO x duration of time = MSP.)

Week 2

Continue addressing biomechanical issues with mobility/corrective exercises; build APO and strength foundation in core, upper body, and lower body; and raise total overload in your MSP workouts. This week will include 2 or 3 days of MO workouts. *Note:* Biomechanics issues aren't solved overnight. Keep working on them over the months.

Week 3

Continue to focus on strength and biomechanical/postural problem areas and raise your MSP efforts by adding weight and time if possible. This week will include 2 or 3 days of MO workouts.

Week 4

Continue to build strength, raise your APO, and add time to your MSP efforts. This week will include 2 or 3 days of MO workouts.

CALENDAR 2 (WEEKS 5 TO 8): IMPROVE STRENGTH, APO, AND MSP

	SUNDAY	MONDAY	TUESDAY	
WEEK 5	Off day, cross-train, or easy short spin	Maximum Overload workout with 2-minute MSP with heavier weight	Easy LSD ride	
WEEK 6	Off day, cross-train, or easy short spin	Maximum Overload workout with 2-minute MSP and heavier weight	Easy LSD ride	
WEEK 7	Off day, cross-train, or easy short spin	Maximum Overload workout with 2-minute MSP and heavier weight	Easy LSD ride	
WEEK 8	Off day, cross-train, or easy short spin	Maximum Overload workout with 2-minute MSP and heavier weight	Easy LSD ride	

Weeks 5 to 8:
Improve Strength, APO, and MSP

Goal: Continue to work on improving strength, but now, if possible, work on improving your APO and MSP efforts. This week will include 2 days of MO workouts, alternating between long and short workouts, with Monday being the MSP workout and Wednesday the APO test. This will leave you fresher for a hard ride on the weekend.

Wednesday will utilize a PAP (postactivation potentiation) workout—see Chapter 6—that stacks an interval after the MO weight workout.

Two days of MSP is pretty brutal.

WEDNESDAY	THURSDAY	FRIDAY	SATURDAY
PAP workout: MO + intervals, with APO test but no MSP walking-lunge workout	Tempo/LSD ride or easy cross-training day	Active recovery ride	Alternative MO workout or big long aerobic ride
PAP workout: MO + intervals, with APO test but no MSP walking-lunge workout	Tempo/LSD ride or easy cross-training day	Active recovery ride	Alternative MO workout or big long aerobic ride
PAP workout: MO + intervals, with APO test but no MSP walking-lunge workout	Tempo/LSD ride or easy cross-training day	Active recovery ride	The big one: race, century ride, or any long event
PAP workout: MO + intervals, with APO test but no MSP walking-lunge workout	Tempo/LSD ride or easy cross-training day	Active recovery ride	The big one: race, century ride, or any long event

Week 5

Continue to work on improving strength, but now if possible add more weight to your MSP efforts. This week will include 2 days of MO workouts, alternating between heavy and light workouts, with Monday being the MSP workout and Wednesday the APO test, plus intervals. This will leave you fresher for a hard ride on the weekend.

If your MSP walking-lunge weight is 25 pounds, now's the time to test to see if you can do 30 or 35 pounds. These efforts are not for time. You rest for full recovery between each one.

Week 6

Work on establishing max lifts on your strength exercises. Think about areas that need work and focus more on extending the time of Monday's MSP workouts. Continue to do 2 MO days, with Wednesday still being the APO test, plus intervals.

Week 7

You are probably within 10 percent of your maximum strength, but will continue to add more time to your MSP efforts. Do 2 MO, with the Monday MSP effort and the APO test on Wednesday, plus intervals.

Week 8

Retest your APO to bump up your weight while still maintaining the same velocity. Stay with your strength maintenance, focusing on the primary lifts. Maintain the Monday MSP workout and the Wednesday APO test, plus intervals.

Weeks 9 to 12: Maintain Strength and Extend MSP Duration

Although still part of your off-season training, the third month of Maximum Overload reprioritizes your schedule as your strength and power approach their potential and the regular riding season beckons. After all, we're not trying to turn you into a weight lifter, but a more powerful rider. After 8 weeks, with the majority of your strength and power gains now made, you drop to one Maximum Overload workout per week (on Mondays). As you shift to more riding time in Weeks 9 to 12, your goal in the gym is try to hold your APO for a longer period of time; i.e., raise your sustainable power, by extending your MSP workout duration from 2 to 3 to 4 minutes. These gains in power will have the effect of giving you bigger overloads on the bike, so your bike training will have greater training value—almost turning your bike into a weight machine on wheels.

Week 9

Do an MO workout on Monday to maintain your strength while extending your MSP duration to 2:30 or 3 minutes. Only add a Wednesday MO if you don't do a hard on-the-bike tempo, hill climb, or interval session that day.

Week 10

Continue strength maintenance and extending your MSP duration to 3 minutes or 3:30 with the Monday MO workout. Your primary goal now is to add more time.

Weeks 11 and 12

Do one early-week MO workout. This lets you use your improved pedaling power in the subsequent on-the-road work.

CALENDAR 3 (WEEKS 9 TO 12): MAINTAIN STRENGTH AND EXTEND MSP DURATION

	SUNDAY	MONDAY	TUESDAY	
WEEK 9	Off day, cross-train, or easy short spin	Maximum Overload workout with MSP focused on maintaining weight and extend time to 2:30 or 3 minutes	Easy LSD ride	
WEEK 10	Off day, cross-train, or easy short spin	Maximum Overload workout with MSP focused on maintaining weight and extend time to 3:00 or 3:30	Easy LSD ride	
WEEK 11	Off day, cross-train, or easy short spin	Maximum Overload workout with MSP focused on maintaining weight and extend time to 3:30 or 4 minutes	Easy LSD ride	
WEEK 12	Off day, cross-train, or easy short spin	Maximum Overload workout with MSP focused on maintaining weight and raising time to 4 minutes	Easy LSD ride	

WEEKLY IN-SEASON TRAINING OVERVIEW

While everyone follows a personalized in-season training program and can adapt a Maximum Overload into it as he or she sees fit, two conditions must apply.

1. You must bookend MO with easy training days—the former to assure that you'll be fresh for the rigors of

WEDNESDAY	THURSDAY	FRIDAY	SATURDAY
Short (1- to 2-hour) high-intensity tempo ride, hill climbing, or intervals	Long (2- to 3-hour) tempo/ LSD ride or easy cross-training day	1-hour active recovery ride or spinning	The big one: race, century ride, or any long event
Short (1- to 2-hour) high-intensity tempo ride, hill climbing, or intervals	Long (2- to 3-hour) tempo/LSD ride or easy cross-training day	1-hour active recovery ride or spinning	The big one: race, century ride, or any long event
Short (1- to 2-hour) high-intensity tempo ride, hill climbing, or intervals	Long (2- to 3-hour) tempo/LSD ride or easy cross-training day	1-hour active recovery ride or spinning	The big one: race, century ride, or any long event
Short (1- to 2-hour) high-intensity tempo ride, hill climbing, or intervals	Long (2- to 3-hour) tempo/LSD ride or easy cross-training day	1-hour active recovery ride or spinning	The big one: race, century ride, or any long event

weight training and the latter to recover from it. Despite being in season, this is not a watered-down Maximum Overload workout, but a heavy-weight, full-blown effort topped off with a monster MSP test. That's because you want to continue to maintain or even build MSP all season long. Remember, as you stay strong, others are wearing out.

2. You should try to do the Maximum Overload workout early in the week (certainly not any later than Wednesday) in order to stay fresh for the big rides and races on the weekend. This contrasts with the more frequent MO schedule in the off-season, when it's not as important to have fresh legs on the weekend.

IN-SEASON SCHEDULE: MAINTAIN STRENGTH AND MSP

SUNDAY	Off day, cross-train, or easy short spin
MONDAY	Maximum Overload workout with heavy deadlifts and full 3- to 4-minute MSP test.
TUESDAY	Easy LSD ride
WEDNESDAY	Group ride/spin class
THURSDAY	Rest day or easy tempo ride
FRIDAY	Active recovery ride or cross-training
SATURDAY	Big ride—race or century

WHEN IN DOUBT, REMEMBER THIS: GO HARD, GO EASY

Maximizing the sustainable power of
Maximum Overload with intervals, LSD, and
staying out of the Black Hole

Rest is underrated.

In the gym and on the bike, endurance athletes simply don't get enough rest. When it comes to fitness, they think rest has no place and that going slow and "taking it easy" is a sign of laziness. After all, they work out to get a workout. Rest is what you do when you're 90, right?

Wrong. Rest is a key element to workouts—before, during and afterward. It's essential if you want to get better. And that goes for all aspects of the comprehensive Maximum Overload training plan, from the weight lifting to the complementary tried-and-true on-the-bike training methods that we all know and love: intervals and long slow distance (LSD) training.

Rest is a key element in Maximum Overload—remember "the rest between the reps" of the weight lifting? Rest plays a key role in the sequential order of the mix of day-to-day workouts. The mandatory rest period between intervals lets you recover and keep the exercises at maximal intensity. A key purpose of LSD training is active rest and recovery from the previous day's hard workout; push LSD too hard and you enter the "Black Hole," a deleterious training zone that can overtrain you and wreck the fat-burning engine LSD is designed to help build.

So to build Maximum Sustainable Power (MSP), you have to maximize the effectiveness of all your workouts, in the gym and on the road—and rest is crucial. Shortcut the rest, and you will sabotage your hard work.

Rest, rest, rest. Remember that the epiphany that led Jacques DeVore to Maximum Overload was that a brief pause or rest is what ultimately allows you to lift more reps of heavy weights and amass a far greater cumulative total of weight.

With rest being as important to training as hard work, here's a simple formula that every endurance athlete should commit to memory if he/she wants to improve or just stay fit: **Go hard, then go easy.**

Rest seems like the easy part of this sentence. But as you'll soon see, it's not so easy to get that rest.

SECTION 1: MAXIMUM OVERLOAD INTERVALS

Intervals, the all-out wind sprints that every former high-school runner, basketball player, and football player recalls with dread, are short, high-speed, high-intensity efforts that amplify and fine-tune your gym-built, ever-more-powerful Maximum Overload body for the road. In a fast 20-minute workout done once a week (which is all most people can handle), they complement Maximum Overload in a very sport-specific way, including upgrades to your speed, structural integrity, endurance, oxygen-processing capability, and lactic-acid buffering ability.

Intervals help you lose weight, due to an hours-long rise in your metabolism, which burns fat.

Intervals work and improve all three energy/fuel-burning systems utilized in any type of human movement: the ATP-PC system, the "drag-racing" engine that supports sub-12-second all-out efforts; the anaerobic glycolytic system, the "V8" engine that takes over in hard, long-sprint efforts 12 to 30 seconds long; and even, surprisingly, the aerobic system's highly oxygen- and fat-dependent economy-car engine.

In addition, numerous studies (such as this one in *Sports Medicine*[1]) have suggested that high-intensity exercise like sprints and weight training can even cause an antiaging effect, due to a temporary boost in human growth hormone (HGH) and testosterone (T), which both drop off radically with age. (Lengthy efforts like cycling stage races, centuries, and even too-long gym sessions can depress hormone levels and raise cortisol, a hormone that breaks down body tissues.)

While you can't prepare your body for a road race or a century ride on intervals alone—mainly because they don't improve your fat-burning machinery and oxygen utilization like LSD does, don't give your body enough time on the road to get used to the stresses of long miles, and are so hard that you shouldn't really do more than one session a week—intervals also have significant endurance benefits. Alarmed by the interval's sudden anaerobic demands on the body, your central nervous system speeds up its information processing and rapidly pushes your VO_2 max (maximal oxygen-delivery capability) closer to its genetic limit. It sends orders to build new capillaries, make more mitochondria, boost stronger lungs and heart, and create a higher anaerobic threshold, so you can suck in more oxygen to go faster without building up lactic acid (an oxygen-debt by-product, which some researchers see as trash and others as fuel, that an interval-trained body can burn very efficiently).

All told, regular interval sessions can accomplish amazing things. A 2006 study at Canada's McMaster University found that cyclists doing interval training developed the same fitness in 20 minutes a day as others riding at a moderate pace for 2 hours—six times longer![2]

What that means is that hard, fast anaerobic efforts like intervals give you aerobic and anaerobic benefits at the same time. Steady-paced LSD training only gives you aerobic. Intervals multitask.

Intervals even work for very high-level athletes. A 2005 study at New Zealand's Waikato Institute of Technology found that intervals even sped up bike racers in midseason form.[3] Eight to 12 sessions gave test subjects power gains of 8.7 percent for 1 kilometer and 8.1 percent for 4 kilometers over a control group of noninterval racers.

To maximize performance benefits from intervals, think quality, not quantity. DeVore doesn't think you can hold quality in more than 6 to 8 intervals. Interval guru Phil Campbell, inventor of the popular Sprint 8 protocol found in his book *Ready, Set, Go! Synergy Fitness*, says, "If you can do more than 8 intervals, you aren't trying hard enough." To push hard, come in rested. Doing intervals prefatigued, such as the day after a Maximum Overload gym workout, will cause submaximal efforts and risk bad form and injuries.

According to renowned sports scientist Tudor O. Bompa,[4] intervals can be a good gauge of fatigue. If your feet feel slow in circling the pedals and the first sprints lack their usual quickness, stop the workout—it means your fast-twitch fibers (which fatigue quicker than endurance-oriented slow-twitch fibers) need a rest. Even if you do manage fast sprints while fatigued, Bompa says you don't get credit for them, as your beat-up body can't process the information well. Although sloppy intervals burn calories, they risk injury and don't do a good job grooving the neuromuscular pathways and hormonal response that'll make you a faster, more coordinated athlete. Again, the key is rest. If your fitness is lacking, do 3 or 4 intervals at first and then build up.

Intervals Strategy

Not surprisingly, DeVore's strategy on intervals mirrors his Maximum Overload protocol for weights: Establish a baseline

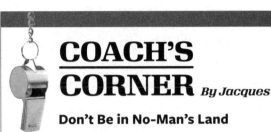

COACH'S CORNER *By Jacques*

Don't Be in No-Man's Land

When I was at the Olympic Training Center in El Cajon, California, going through the Expert USA Cycling certification program in 2001, we had a presenter who discussed the use of power meters. At the time, power was a relatively new concept left more to pros and high-level amateurs. Coming to cycling with a background in strength and conditioning, I raised my hand and asked a question.

"Are you monitoring total volume of time at different levels of power to see the impact on overall performance?" In other words, how much time was spent at 150, 200, or 500 watts?

The answer surprised me: "I don't know. I've never thought about that."

I bit my tongue—because I was utterly shocked. This valuable metric, this essential measure of how much work was actually being done, was being ignored, was being made useless! You need to measure overload accurately to get the desired performance adaptation.

When it came to overloads and adaptations with power, the coaches were not seeing the whole picture.

In weight lifting, the total amount of volume and intensity is important. You can lift a 50-pound weight 10 times or lift 250 pounds twice. The total of both is 500 pounds—but the two workouts are obviously very different. The stresses on your muscles—the overloads—might be minimal at 50 pounds and maximal at 250 pounds. To make someone stronger and more powerful, you have to use high overloads, not light or medium

of distance and/or mph by doing 6 or 7 "reps" (30-second sprints followed by 2 minutes of rest) to failure, then break that set into 15-second mini-sets that allow you to get in a bigger total overload at high intensity.

The gap between maximum power output on an inter-

ones, and you have to know how much volume you're doing to be able to figure out what's working. The same thing goes for power training on the bike.

You do not want to be in No Man's Land—the place where most cyclists spend way too much of their training time. No Man's Land is when you're riding too hard for recovery and not hard enough for an overload. The same thing can occur in the gym.

When I worked with Dave Zabriskie in the fall of 2012, I was not only his strength coach, but also his cycling coach. I was able to monitor his power on the bike and observe how the Maximum Overload training was impacting his sustainable power performance. Was he bumping up his maximum power output and sustaining greater amounts of power for longer periods of time, our goals? We were aiming for the power "gold standard"—a power-to-weight ratio of 5 to 6 watts per kilogram of body weight—and we wanted him to hold it as long as possible.

Believe me—there was no No Man's Land in Zabriskie's training. With me, he worked out heavier and harder than he ever had before—on the bike as well as in the gym. We gave him huge overloads because we wanted his body to send loud-and-clear signals to his DNA to make improvements and to make them fast. It worked. His power-to-weight ratio rose to 5-plus watts per kilo. His power jumped by 15 percent in 4 months—unheard of for a professionally trained athlete. It even caught me by surprise. But it was a good lesson in the power of pushing a maximum overload—not a submaximum overload—and knowing exactly how big it is and how often you're doing it.

val and normal riding is huge and may explain why some studies show that a relative handful of intervals can have a pronounced impact on the fitness of both trained and untrained cyclists. While pros can typically hold 300 to 400-plus watts of power for 20 minutes (a gold standard known as "functional threshold power"), they put out 1,800+ watts of maximum power in a 15-second sprint. Amateurs can hold 200 to 300 watts for 20 minutes and put out 1,000 watts of power in a 15-second interval. Jolting your system with five or six times its "regular" wattage is a radical overload that can push up your 20-minute functional threshold wattage. Maximum Overload's mini-set scheme can almost double your cumulative interval time.

Here's how to set up a standard interval workout and its Maximum Overload variant.

First, get your baseline.

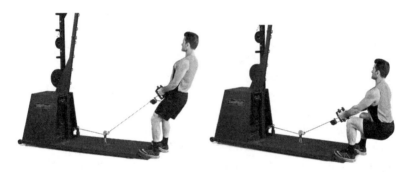

Here, the athlete does intervals using a VersaPulley, a specialized machine DeVore uses in his gym.

The best way to measure your overload is with wattage numbers from a power meter. But if you don't have one, you can also use distance (with a landmark like a mailbox as a goal) or average mph from a bike computer over a designated distance. With each session, note the gear and cadence you use.

Some interval programs use eight intervals, but DeVore likes six for most people, thinking that a seventh and eighth will be poor quality submaximal efforts (which yield submaximal results). You want good quality on all these balls-out, leave-nothing-on-the-table efforts; once you reach failure—the point of fatigue—stop. The first three intervals typically won't be a struggle because you're fresh, have a lot of oxygen floating around your system, and will be refreshed by the 2-minute rest. Number three will often be the best one. But after that, sprints four, five, and six will be tougher; 2 minutes of rest won't seem like enough. You can typically maintain quality through six. Only superfit people should push it to eight.

Why the 30-second duration for the intervals? DeVore has found that 30-second intervals are not too short and not too long. "You can maintain maximum power output to 30 seconds," he says. "From 30 seconds to a minute, your power drops off, moving you into the glycolytic energy system. You want to stay in the ATP zone."

Also, mentally, 30 seconds do not demoralize you like 45 or 60 do. You can do the first 20 seconds "pretty easily," he says, "then hang on for the last 10."

Once you have your 6 x 30-second baseline, you can kick it up a notch by applying the Maximum Overload template: Break the 30-second intervals into 15-second mini-sets to raise the cumulative overload at your higher output and improve MSP. DeVore recommends this three-set pattern:

Set 1: 15-sec. interval + 15-sec. rest. Repeat for 3 min. Total intervals = 6

Set 2: 15-sec. interval + 10-sec. rest. Repeat for 3 min. Total intervals = 7

Set 3:   15-sec. interval + 5-sec. rest. Repeat for 3 min. Total intervals = 9

Rest for 3 or 4 minutes between sets; you want to be fully recovered. Total time for the workout, including a 5-minute warm-up, is 20 minutes. Total intervals at maximum power output = 22. Bottom line: In the same 20-minute workout time, the 15-second scheme gives you more total time at all-out wattage ($5\frac{1}{2}$ minutes) than with the 30-second intervals (3 minutes). Of course, lowering your heart-rate during the 15-, 10-, and 5-second rests won't be easy. If so, go back to the simpler 8 x 30 scheme.

Once you've done these, your goal is to constantly keep extending the distance that you cover in the 15 seconds—i.e., do 'em faster, which means your power is going up.

DeVore recommends doing one interval session a week, alternating between the 30-second and 15-second schemes. One supports the other. It's the same reason why Maximum Overload's weight-training workouts alternate between the Monday MSP workout (with 40 to 90+ steps) and the Wednesday APO—absolute power output—test (with one to three 12-step efforts). The former really fries you; the latter will leave you fresher for the big Saturday ride or race.

You can perform Maximum Overload cycling intervals on the road, at home on a bike trainer, and at the gym on a spin bike or Lifecycle. Cyclists can also get great interval benefits by cross-training with running or stair-climbing, or by doing VersaClimber and elliptical-machine intervals, which offer important posture and bone-building benefits for cyclists (see Chapter 8) due to their upright, weight-bearing stance.

Pressed for Time? Try PAP

If you want to do intervals, but don't want to devote a sole workout to them, try what Bompa calls "Post-Activation Potentiation" (PAP), which conveniently piggybacks an interval session on top of a Maximum Overload workout. In fact, PAP might even improve your intervals. The weight lifting essentially warms you up, stimulating the central nervous system and the muscle fiber neurons for high-intensity work and priming you for a better-than-normal interval workout. That way, PAP turns sprints into supersprints and accelerates their benefits. Muscles stay warm and "optimized" for 5 to 30 minutes after the strength workout, so it behooves you to do sprints without delay. DeVore used PAP frequently with Dave Zabriskie because both felt it worked.

For pure time savings, PAP can't be beat. In a fast-paced hour (consisting of a 40-minute Maximum Overload workout and 20 minutes of sprints) you knock off two hard, intense workouts at once that can share recovery on the following day. That saves you an extra workout day or rest day—time you can spend with the family, go out to dinner, or even take a ride. But for the sake of recovery, make it an easy one.

SECTION 2: THE HARD/EASY PARADIGM, LSD, AND THE EVIL BLACK HOLE

It's worth repeating: If you forget everything about Maximum Overload and interval training—the reps, the math, the progressions, the exercises, the periodization—just remember four words: **Go hard, go easy.** That framework is the key to athletic success, especially for endurance.

It's really that simple: Work out hard one day, and work out easy the next. Never do two hard days in a row (unless it is designed for a big overload or is a stage race when fitness is required at a high level).

Whether your sport is bodybuilding or basketball or cycling, most bodies need at least 48 hours of recovery after hard strength and cardio workouts to repair and improve their muscles' fast-twitch fibers, which do the brunt of any high-intensity work. Back-to-back hard training days restress your already-stressed muscles before they are fully recovered from the first workout—a recipe for injuries, muscle soreness, fatigue, and psychological burnout. (That's one of the reasons why DeVore is wary of relentless high-intensity programs like CrossFit, which he believes lead to injuries—"and use random choices in weight that may be too light or too heavy to build Maximum Sustainable Power, anyway," he says—although he has occasionally designed multiple-day overloads to simulate stage races.) The simple hard/easy paradigm avoids overtraining and keeps you fit, healthy, and improving.

There are several ways to get this necessary "easy" workout. You could kick back and watch TV all day. Better, you could do a nonstressful cross-training activity like hiking, golf, or some easy swimming.

Or even better for a cyclist, you could ride. Ride easy and consistently, staying aerobic with a low heart rate. There's a name for it: LSD—long slow distance.

Most cyclists know about LSD. It's a great way to upgrade the long-distance infrastructure—joints, bones, and muscles—that you'll need for long hours in the unusual cycling position. And it serves as a physical and psychological break from the rigors of hard training; think of it as a carefree reward for all your hard work.

But what people don't know about LSD is that it is the sole element of your cycling training you absolutely must get right. You can be somewhat imprecise while doing weight lifting and intervals and still get some of the benefit. But pushing the pace too fast by just a few heartbeats for too long while doing LSD will compromise your recovery and its most crucial benefit: supercharging your engine to utilize more fat as fuel so you can ride strong all day long.

LSD optimizes you for endurance due to these interrelated benefits.

- **Improved slow-twitch muscle fibers,** which specialize in endurance (weights and intervals build only fast-twitch fibers)
- **More high-mileage mitochondria** (the muscles' tiny intercellular engines densely packed in slow-twitch fibers). LSD alters them to burn a higher percentage of fat for fuel. (All fuel mixes consist of both carbs and fat.)
- **Bigger pipeline to fat,** which your body has an unlimited supply of (done with the help of a higher-fat/low-carb diet—see Chapter 7)
- **Greater oxygen supply.** Fat requires O_2 to burn. By staying aerobic, you supply a lot more of it.
- **Support for the more intense intervals.** This may be counterintuitive, but you recover more quickly after an interval session if you have a good aerobic base.

Taken together, these changes transform you into a "fat-burning beast" primed for long miles and long life. (Credit the term to paleo guru Mark Sisson; see Chapter 7.) Fat is an ideal long-haul fuel. You have a virtually unlimited supply of it, so you require no major refueling during an event, and it's a much cleaner-burning fuel than sugar/carb-based glycogen, leaving less hormonal disturbance, unhealthy cellular trash, and oxidation in its wake. Endurance athletes who have trained themselves to fuel up on extremely high percentages of fat report that they were able to eat much less during the event—particularly sugary carbs—and suffer less gastric distress as a result.

The upshot: With the low-carb diet putting more and better fuel into your engine and LSD rebuilding and enlarging the engine itself, you're healthier and optimized for endurance. That means more mileage and more speed at less effort.

Given all the above, LSD seems to be a tailor-made complement to the Maximum Overload plan.

There's a big caveat, however: As we said earlier, you have to get it right. You can't let LSD become non-LSD, or you'll wreck the benefits. You have to keep the recovery day pure. Unfortunately, on a bike, that's not as easy as it sounds.

After all, people forget. We often go all or nothing. We're type A. We start off easy, but . . . can't resist hammering out of the saddle on the first climb or shifting into the big ring. It's hard not to try to keep up when your friends surge. Before you know it, you're not doing a restful, easy ride anymore. By leaving the "easy" heart-rate zone and going anaerobic, you're burning more sugar/less fat, not improving your slow-twitch fibers, compromising your recovery, short-circuiting the adaptations from the hard workouts, and breaking your muscles down again before they have a chance to fully build themselves back up. Do this often enough and you end up sore all the time, fatigued, riding poorly, and overtrained.

Interestingly, you don't have to blast up a monster hill with lungs heaving to wreck your recovery. Hard efforts just into the anaerobic heart-rate zone will do it, too—your subconscious acceleration over the freeway overpasses in an otherwise flat route, pushing just hard enough to where you can't quite speak in full sentences, your spin class. Many people—maybe most—unwittingly spend all their "recovery" rides in this sort-of-hard zone, which they think is okay because it's not really a hard effort. But just the same, it's wrecking their recovery.

It's called the Black Hole.

The Black Hole is a pace that is too hard for recovery but not hard enough for an overload. Think of it, in Maximum Overload terms, as being submaximal; not a big enough overload to force your body to adapt, but still taxing. The Black Hole is insidious, tricking you into going too fast without knowing it. It's a narrow heart-rate zone, just seven or eight heartbeats wide, that starts when you switch from aerobic to anaerobic metabolism. It's an alluring place to camp in for most of us, because it's not hellishly hard like an interval, but just hard enough to make you feel like you got in a real workout. In fact, the Black Hole is such a satisfying place to train in that most people stay in it day after day, year after year: It's their daily run or ride.

But if you want the hard work of your Maximum Overload training to pay off fully, stay out of the Black Hole.

THE FAT-BURNING ENGINE, EXPLAINED

The "engine" in "fat-burning engine" refers to your muscles, their supporting nerve and circulatory systems, and two things we've all heard of but only sort of understand: slow-twitch muscles and mitochondria.

Muscles are made up of several different types of muscle fibers, including slow-twitch (or type I) fibers that handle slower, aerobic activities like standing, walking, and even marathon-length running, and fast-twitch fibers (type IIA, X, and B) that handle faster, more explosive activities like 20-minute tempo runs, sprints, and 1-rep deadlifts respectively. Long and smooth, slow-twitch fibers are the only ones that run on fat; they get their name from their slow contractions and high fatigue resistance. Shorter and bulkier, fast-twitch fibers contract fast and are fueled by nonfat fuels like glycogen. Of course, slow-twitch is the go-to LSD endurance fiber because it can run all day on your body's virtually unlimited fat supply.

Slow-twitch fibers are colored red because they are jam-packed with red-hued mitochondria, microscopic motors within the muscle cells. Fast-twitch type IIA fibers have less mitochondria, but still a lot, and therefore are also red. The other fast-twitch fibers are white in color because they have much less mitochondria. Every cell in every organism has at least one mitochondrion; the specialized cells of the liver are jammed with 1,000 to 2,000 of them. Slow-twitch fibers are the most mitochondria-dense muscle fibers.

Like the cylinders in a car engine, mitochondria suck in oxygen, ignite fuel, and create energy that runs the cell. The more mito-

If you haven't heard of the Black Hole, don't be surprised. It's been around forever, but didn't have a name until an international team of sports researchers identified it in 2007 in an eye-opening survey of the training habits of elite endurance athletes.[5]

chondria you have and the more efficient your mitochondria is, the more weight you can lift, speed you can run, and miles you can go. One way to add to their efficiency is by switching to a low-carb diet; mitochondria naturally burn fatty acids cleaner than they burn carbohydrates, in the process producing fewer free radicals and an anti-inflammatory effect. And, of course, because mitochondria adapt to stress just like the muscles they inhabit, another way to make them multiply and improve is exercise—especially LSD training. That's because the slow-twitch fibers that handle LSD are so jammed with mitochondria.

As the LSD training effect upgrades your blood vessels, lungs, and heart along with your mitochondria, every heartbeat will provide more oxygen and nutrients and faster removal of carbon dioxide and lactate. That's why, through training, you'll eventually be going faster at the same heart rate.

LSD is not the only way to jack up your mitochondrial density. Strength training, done in concert with LSD, enhances the effect. Intervals do it, too, and in half the time of LSD alone. So why not just use intervals and skip LSD? Well, since intervals burn carbs, they don't optimize mitochondria for fat-burning like LSD does, so they'll only get you in shape for shorter runs and tris under an hour long. Also, intervals have a high injury risk.

LSD isn't perfect, as it is catabolic (does not build or even maintain muscle) and produces little new mitochondria when you do it for over an hour. But there's no getting around it: For long-distance events, nothing is more effective for building up your endurance machinery than low-heart-rate LSD training.

The study leaders, exercise scientists Jonathan-Esteve Lanos of the European University of Madrid, Carl Foster of the University of Wisconsin at La Crosse, and Stephen Seiler, an American teaching at Agder University College in Kristiansand, Norway, discovered that those who spent the most

training time in the Black Hole had the worst race performances and most injuries, while those with the smallest time
in the Black Hole got healthier and faster. They found that
the best performances came out of training that included
8 to 10 percent intervals, 80 to 85 percent LSD, and the
remainder in the Black Hole, which was usually done going in

AT THE RACES

In his own words, here's what happened when one of a trio
of Cat 2 and Cat 3 racers ranging in age from their 30s to
their 50s trained with Maximum Overload.

DAVID BAAR

*"My climbing has never felt as
awesome"*

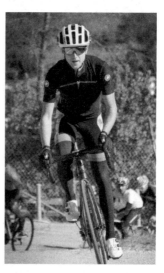

Age: 30

Occupation: Data analyst

Residence: Los Angeles

Level: Category 2 racer

Accomplishment: Raised 1-minute
time-trial wattage by 5 percent in
3 weeks of training and completed
85-kilometer 3,275-meter Taiwan
KOM Challenge

After training with Jacques for 2 months now, I'm seriously
impressed by my progress. I would describe myself as the
typical traditional cyclist who loves to climb and hence is
almost "scared" of lifting weights. However, I do have an open
mind, and once I was introduced to Jacques' Maximum Overload

and out of intervals. Their conclusion: Better recovery, *not* additional hard efforts, led to better performance.

Incidentally, the name "Black Hole" appears nowhere in the study. It's not "scientific" enough to put in a research paper; it's just shorthand between PhDs. It was coined by Seiler, who mentioned the term to this book's coauthor in a

method, I knew that if I wanted to break the stagnation of the last year and get to a new level, I had to try it out.

The immediate results were amazing. After 3 weeks, I set a new watts/kg personal best for a 1-minute effort, 5 percent higher than what I tested just the weekend before Jacques started my training. The next eye-opener was another 3 weeks later, when I lined up for the Taiwan KOM Challenge, which features probably one of the toughest climbs on this planet. Continuously climbing from sea level to 3,275 meters, the last 10 kilometers are the real test of mental and physical fitness. This last stretch of the 85-kilometer climb features gradients as high as 27 percent and averages around 15 percent. It was brutal and beautiful at the same time. The best part was the confidence I gained after I went over the first steeper part and realized that after 4 hours of climbing, the power was still there to push through, even if it was getting steeper and steeper. This was new to me, and I solely attribute that to the Maximum Overload approach, as that is exactly what we focused on.

After this realization, I couldn't wait to get back to Los Angeles and to continue my training with Jacques in preparation for the 2017 season. If the first 6 weeks are an indicator, it should definitely be a real good one. At this point, I'm 2 months into my training and the improvements occurred exactly as predicted by Jacques: Power is up, body weight remains the same, and climbing never felt as awesome!

2010 *Outside* magazine article.[6] An astronomy enthusiast, Seiler said that this deleterious training zone was analogous to the Black Hole in space, which has an awesome gravitational pull that he says "sucks everything in." Basically, the not-too-hard/not-too-easy heart-rate zone sucks slow cyclists into going too fast and fast cyclists into going too slow. In Maximum Overload speak, either way you look at the Black Hole, it's submaximal.

"This pace makes you think you're working hard," says Seiler, "but it's actually too easy to force your body to get fitter and too hard to allow it to recover. To get better as an athlete, you have to go really hard and really easy and stay out of the in-between."

The Black Hole is located in a tiny sliver of heart rate about seven beats wide between LSD and high-intensity training and does not give you the benefits of either. It starts at a metabolic breakpoint called "threshold"—the point where recovery ends, lactate levels start to rise, and anaerobic metabolism begins. Just over the line, you start to breathe harder to get more oxygen in, but it's still easy enough that you don't notice it . . . and you push it even more.

Translating threshold to heart-rate numbers you can use, your Black Hole would be the narrow zone between 100 and 105 percent of threshold. So, if your threshold is 150 beats per minute (bpm), your Black Hole would be 150 to 157.5 bpm. All the numbers will change with your fitness level.

Sticking with the 150 bpm threshold here, the impact of moving just from 148 bpm to 152 bpm would be surprisingly dramatic. Switching from a pure aerobics system, where

DON'T BE LIKE ERIC

While the hard/easy paradigm is the rule for 99 percent of us, certain genetically gifted world-class athletes can violate it sometimes, managing to work out hard all the time without a break with great success. But don't be too impressed. "They are not examples to be emulated," warns Carl Foster, who cites the case of speed-skating star (and future elite cyclist) Eric Heiden, who won five of five possible speed-skating gold medals at the 1980 Olympic Games—and thereby made life miserable for the next generation of skaters.

In sports, as in life, everyone copies the greats. "The trouble was that Heiden's physiology was unique—he could train hard every day," says Foster. "The average guy—even the average world-class athlete—can't, requiring at least 48 hours (not just 24) to recover from a hard workout." That's why Bonnie Blair (a four-time Olympian who won five speed-skating gold medals and a bronze from 1984 to 1994) changed coaches and stopped talking to Foster when she began suffering less-than-optimal results in her ramp-up to the 1992 Olympics.

"She had a fairly normal physiology," explains Foster. "She needed more rest than the coaches were giving her." She took it, and soon she was winning again.

Years later, she told Foster he'd failed her because he hadn't told the coaches to give her a day off for recovery. "'So what good are you as a physiologist?' she told me," he said. Foster was dumbstruck. He couldn't argue with her.

The takeaway: If you want to improve and are more like Bonnie than Eric (as most of us are), it's best to follow a hard, intense day (or two) with an easy recovery day.

And if you want to avoid injuries, stay excited about your fitness training, and be your best, you must get complete recovery on that recovery day. Otherwise, your body won't get the recharge it needs, and you won't be at full power for your next hard workout.

90 to 95 percent of an endurance athlete's energy is fueled mainly by fat, to a Black Hole pace that burns more sugar, a litany of bad stuff starts to happen: You run out of fuel faster, wreck your recovery, spin off more free radical and cellular trash, etc. And while your brain may not notice this, the body does. Anything over threshold is considered a hard workout by the body, according to Foster. "We think there's a physiological tripwire," he says. "Slip into the Black Hole for a few minutes—or do an interval or two—and the body reads the whole workout as hard. It cancels the LSD's recovery effect."

How to Find the Black Hole

All this leads to the obvious question: If the Black Hole is so hard to detect, how do you identify it? How do you avoid succumbing to its tantalizing allure?

First, find your threshold by taking the talk test: Slowly increase your riding speed while saying the Pledge of Allegiance. At the point you can't say it without panting, look at your heart-rate monitor. That number is your approximate threshold. Then set the heart-rate monitor to beep when you approach that bpm. (If you've got the money and the time, find your threshold by having a training lab analyze fingertip blood samples taken at different intensity levels as you ride a stationary bike.)

SUMMARY

Whether you are a world-class athlete looking for a secret weapon or a couch potato using the Maximum Overload plan to jump-start a healthier life, the same training rules apply: To get better, you have to go really hard on the hard days (Maximum Overload and intervals) and really easy on the easy days (LSD)—and keep out of the middle (the Black Hole).

Those easy LSD days, which help build your aerobic base and your fat-burning machinery and provide recovery, are not as easy as they might seem. Whether you do long or short LSD rides (it's best to match your LSD duration to your event, says DeVore, with multiday stage racers and century riders requiring more than track riders and 45-minute criterium racers), going easy is often the most difficult part of the hard/easy rhythm. Don't be too proud or impatient to take it slow. Studies show that 48 hours of recovery is essential to keeping most people's muscles fresh—and Maximum Overload–honed muscles even fresher. So keep the LSD day pure. LSD is necessary and fun. It builds your fat-burning machinery and gives you a break from weights and sprints as it turbocharges their training effect, leaving you stronger, faster, and better able to hold form at a race from beginning to end. Don't sully the LSD by pushing up into the Black.

Granted, working out in the Black Hole is better than sitting on the couch and is fine for anyone trying to get or stay in shape, but it'll keep ambitious athletes slow and tired. If you want to make the most of your training, stay out of it: You're only going to do LSD a couple times a week in this program. Take it easy—and make the most of it.

Go hard. Go easy. And stay out of the Black Hole.

PERFORMANCE-ENHANCING EATING

The natural-food strategy that'll turn you into a faster, lighter, healthier, longer-riding "fat-burning beast"

Power-to-weight is the key concept in cycling performance. If you raise your ratio, you go faster. Maximum Overload training will raise your power. A natural-food diet, the subject of this chapter, will lower your weight. Do both, and you will fly.

And in addition, you'll be healthier and probably live longer.

A good diet goes by various names nowadays—natural, paleo, primal, ancestral. Jacques DeVore calls it the Real-Food No-Label Diet—no trans fat and processed oils, no engineered food products with 73 ingredients. It's the way your great-grandmother ate—back in the day when, as his great-grandmother once told him, "the only obese people were in the circus."

Although experts say you can't exercise off a bad diet, cyclists keep trying. "Cyclists can be what I call 'horribly fit,'" says DeVore. "After a club ride here in West LA, you'll see MAMILs (a bike-industry acronym meaning "middle-aged men in Lycra") sitting around at the coffee shop, mowing down scones and chai tea lattes. They're fit but unhealthy, with their big bellies and clogged veins. It looks like the pier in San Francisco with all the fat sea lions hanging out, carping at each other."

DeVore saw firsthand the effect of a natural-food diet when he coached Dave "DZ" Zabriskie from 2012 to 2013. The heavy-weight training protocol of Maximum Overload wasn't the only reason why the 6-foot rider dropped his body weight from 168 to 154 pounds and raised his pedal power by a whopping 15 percent in just 4 months. On the advice of paleo-movement leader Mark Sisson, a close friend of DeVore, who wrote the bestselling low-carb diet book *Primal Blueprint* and founded the popular Web site marksdailyapple.com, Zabriskie also changed his diet to include more avocados, coconut oil, eggs, almonds, cashews, chicken breasts, beef jerky, and vegetables—and eliminated most bread, pasta, cake, crackers, and sugary energy bars. In other words, he went primal.

Sisson introduced Zabriskie to DeVore, who linked the new diet to the Maximum Overload plan. Before the weight workouts, Zabriskie was instructed to eat nutrient-dense starchy vegetables like carrots, beets, and brussels sprouts to provide the glycogen that fuels rapid, explosive movements.

Adopting a now-common carb-diet strategy of train low, race high, he trained on the bike in a low-glycogen state (for example, putting less Cytomax in his water bottles) to force his muscles to adapt to fat-burning. Over time, he could ride comfortably for 3 hours without a sugary quick-energy gel like a GU. On long training rides, he also used UCAN Super-starch, a unique long-chain carbohydrate formula designed not to spike insulin, which helped wean him off a high-carb diet while not wrecking his fat utilization (insulin, designed to break down sugar and store it as fat, stops fat-burning). On race day, he topped off his stores of carbohydrates in the morning. The plan worked. DZ felt great at the 2013 Tour of Catalonia.

Mimicking the purportedly healthier eating habits of our hunter-gatherer ancestors, who survived on the big animals they could kill and the berries, nuts, and green veggies they could forage, Zabriskie shunned sugars and man-made refined carbs and ate mainly fat and protein. In the process, he returned to man's natural "factory setting" and became what Sisson calls a "fat-burning beast."

A fat-burning beast is paleo/primal-speak for a person who fuels most of his or her activities not on carbs but on the dense, endless, clean-burning calories of stored body fat—yes, the stuff that pads our bellies, butts, and thighs. For decades, many people thought long hours of slow aerobic training was what was required to teach your body to process fat efficiently, a mighty gram of which holds 9 calories of energy versus just 4.5 calories in a gram of sugar. But Sisson and a growing number of researchers think fat-processing efficiency is mainly a matter of what you eat. If you eat lots of candy bars and tortillas, your amazing flexi-fuel body will get good at using sugar and refined flour. If you eat "good" carbs like lettuce and cauliflower, it'll get good at that. If you're like Alaska's whale-eating Inuit, your body will get along just fine on whale blubber and muscle.

The paleo crowd, which has moved from marginal to mainstream in the last few years, believes the ideal for energy and longevity is a low-carb diet, which is high in fat and protein with a good measure of natural (unprocessed, nongrain) carbs from vegetables. This metabolically efficient mix processes fat into energy easily, leaving no damage or waste products behind in the process. Fat is a near-perfect endurance fuel, burning slowly and powerfully, like heavy logs on a fire. On the other hand, sugar and carbs burn hot and fast, and then they are gone, like straw to flame. The standard American diet is more like straw, as it is low in fat and loaded with man-made food that is inefficient, difficult for the body to process, and ultimately unhealthy. Here's the problem.

While humans are omnivores who can process any food for energy, our huge increase in consumption of three food categories—sugars, grained-based refined carbs like bread, and processed oils—over the last 40 years (thank you, Coca-Cola, Cap'n Crunch, and Pizza Hut)—has overwhelmed a system not designed to ingest them in such large amounts. The body just doesn't know what to do with all of this odd stuff.

As a result, these man-made foods have many negative long- and short-term effects on the body, such as the following:

- Sugars and refined carbs cause inflammation, which is linked to diseases like heart disease, delays in recovery, and oxidation.

- They have an addictive response that causes you to eat more, making you fatter.
- Processed industrial oils like trans fats and partially hydrogenated fats damage your cells at the DNA level and are linked to cancer.
- Canola, corn, soybean, and other polyunsaturated vegetable oils—called "free radicals in a bottle" by some—immediately inflict oxidative damage, which accelerates aging and hampers immune and cardio-vascular function.
- They all stop your body from utilizing body fat.

Preventing fat utilization is exactly what you don't want to happen, because the performance benefits of burning body fat for fuel are too good to pass up. A low-carb paleo diet high in animal/fish fat and protein, nuts, fruit, and non-starchy vegetables transforms you in a good way. It's great for long-term health and is a boon for athletic performance that gives you three major performance upgrades that can make cyclists and other endurance athletes faster—even without Maximum Overload.

The first and most important one deals with a simple math problem: What's bigger: 2,000 or 80,000?

WHY FAT MAKES YOU FASTER

1. **Immensely bigger fuel tank:** On race day, the single biggest limiting factor in a long event is the rela-tively tiny amount of glycogen (a form of carbohy-drate) that can be packed in the muscles and used to fuel movement: about 2,000 calories in the normal

adult male. (Don't count on blood sugar to help much; not much more than 40 calories are floating in a healthy person's bloodstream, according to well-known low-fat author/researcher Stephen Phinney.) While everybody burns a mix of glycogen and fat, there will be problems if the glycogen is used up too quickly. Once the 2,000-calorie glycogen tank goes low, usually in 90 minutes or 2 hours of sustained effort, you bonk. Glycogen rules several vital functions, like running your brain, and when it's low, you get lightheaded—i.e., bonk.

By contrast, everybody has an almost unlimited supply of body fat—as much as 80,000 calories' worth, even on skinny people. If you train your body, through eating fewer carbs and more fat, to become a "fat-burning machine," it'll use more fat and less glycogen, thereby delaying the bonk. Tapping your 80,000-calorie fat-fuel tank more often has other benefits, too: You won't need to refuel with a gel or energy bar every 5 or 10 miles to top off your glycogen tank, as high-carb–eating athletes must do, and you won't suffer gastrointestinal problems at mile 75 from eating sugary stuff all day. A high-carb racer might eat 6,000 in-race calories; a fat-adapted low-carb racer might eat a quarter of that. Running on fat and eating less, you can theoretically go strong all day long.

2. **Weight loss:** Pumping more fatty foods into your diet (which might seem odd at first, given all the misguided propaganda we've been fed over the years

about the evils of fat) actually trains your body to use stored fat as fuel; that's how the weight loss occurs. The body gets good at burning whatever fuel is available to it. So as you force it to switch to burning more fat, it reaches for and gets better at melting excess body fat. The weight loss derived from that automatically raises your power-to-weight ratio and makes you faster—without doing any extra work.

In addition to helping you burn more body fat, a fatty diet motivates you to eat less. That's due to a greater satiety than you get from sugar/carb foods, a lower insulin production, and fewer sugar/carb cravings.

3. **Faster recovery:** You get back to full strength quicker after a hard ride with a fat-protein–based diet because it's packed with more of the nutrients that are used to rebuild muscle, such as protein. Additionally, paleo foods are rich in antioxidants, which generate less inflammation and free radicals than sugar/carbs. For pure efficiency's sake, fat burns "cleaner" than sugar in that it leaves less metabolic junk behind in the mitochondria, the little intracellular engines that produce energy.

It is clear that diet is powerful. A primal diet not only has the potential to improve endurance performance, but it also protects you against some of the negative effects of those endurance miles. Unfortunately, we have no known long-term instance of a pro bike rider successfully using a paleo diet; after using it in the Tour of Catalonia, Dave Zabriskie crashed out early at the 2013 Tour of California with a broken collarbone, then retired before the Tour de France. But several high-level paleo athletes in ultrarunning and triathlon have had impressive success, which they partially but heartily attribute to their diet.

In ultrarunning, Timothy Olson won the prestigious Western States 100 in 2102 and 2013 while following a primal diet, as did Zach Bitter in setting new American 100-mile records in 2013 and 2015. Olson, an Ashland, Oregon, massage therapist, raved about his lack of gastrointestinal stress, a chronic problem for him, his lack of need for food during the race, and his unusually quick recovery—a week instead of a month. Bitter, a Wisconsin schoolteacher, became so good at metabolizing fat that a treadmill study by Jeff Volek found that he was running 7-minute miles on an amazing fuel mix of 98 percent fat and 2 percent carbs. Bitter said that spared him stomachaches, kept him cooler, and allowed him to eat less than normal.

In triathlon, Sami Inkinen and Klemen Rojnik used primal diets to blitz the Hawaii Ironman triathlon with impressive sub-9-hour finishing times. Rojnik, a Slovenian pharmaceutical researcher, took second in the 30–34 age group in 2013 at 8:48:35 (38 minutes faster than the year before) while training about 20 percent less than in past (nonpaleo) years, while Inkinen, a Silicon Valley entrepreneur, took second in his 35–39 age group in 2011 at 8:58:59 on 12 hours of training a week, half that of the average Ironman. Both found they needed shots of carbs during high-intensity efforts like intervals and during the race itself, but much less than in previous Ironman races.

Paleo devotees say they weren't surprised by the success of those four athletes and others like them because their experiences played out exactly as the science had predicted. They had rebuilt their aerobic engines in a new, efficient way: They'd gone from being inefficient carb-burners to extremely efficient fat-burners. They'd changed their diets and stayed with it long enough—at least a year or two—to alter their systems to the point where they could utilize fat as their overwhelming source of fuel even at very high speeds. Inkinen guessed that he'd increased the size and efficiency of his aerobic engine—i.e., the density and ability of his muscles' mitochondria to process fat into energy—to the point where they allowed him to "double or triple" the maximum amount of fat he could process for fuel per hour. That translated directly to speed since he could "maintain a higher intensity almost indefinitely" during the race. That's why, as a group, these athletes represent a huge paradigm shift.

Although we don't purport to be experts in all things paleo, we predict that within a decade the best endurance athletes—pros and amateurs alike—will all be paleo. Paleo diets will be the rule—not the exception—for endurance sports, due to sheer competition. Because if you want to keep up with the Olsons and the Rojniks of the world, you'll have to eat like them.

Another reason primal eating will dominate is career longevity. The sheer healthiness of a high-fat/low-carb diet helps mitigate the stresses of mega-miles, keeping you competitive at a time when your nonprimal peers are heading for the rocking chairs.

HOW FOOD SHAPES YOUR AEROBIC ENGINE

Food, not training, builds the healthiest and best-performing fat-burning infrastructure, according to paleo leaders like Sisson. Or to put it more techy: The physiological processes set in motion by a low-carb/high-fat diet literally force the development of an efficient fat-burning engine in a way that training alone can't.

Your body is programmed for survival. It'll use any food for energy. If you take away carbs and give the body more protein and fat, it'll quickly get used to metabolizing more fat as its primary fuel. In fact, according to Harvard instructor Emily Deans, MD, writing in *Evolutionary Psychiatry*, while the body has some essential requirements for protein and fat, it doesn't actually need carbs to live. Our bodies can turn protein into glucose through a process known as *gluconeogenesis*. So while "we would die without eating at least some fat and at least some protein, we can live quite happily while consuming no carbohydrates at all," she says. "That's not saying there aren't some disadvantages or side effects to a so-called 'zero-carb' diet, but it won't cause the massive health problems and death that consuming zero-fat or zero-protein diet would."

Teaching your body to use fat as its primary fuel and spare the little carbohydrates it has, a process Sisson calls "fuel repartitioning," comes down to mitochondria, the tiny engines within each cells that give the muscles the energy to move. Motivated by the ingestion of additional fat, your muscles not only will build more mitochondria, but will also build them better at burning fat. Fat burns cleaner than glycogen, leaving behind fewer pieces of chemical trash and oxidation to hinder recovery and long-term health. "Essentially, you're transforming your 4-cylinder, pollution-spewing, carb-fueled engine into a squeaky-clean, 6-cylinder fat-burning machine," Sisson says. "That's possible because mitochondria are the only structures within the body that have their own DNA and therefore are uniquely adept at changing and multiplying rapidly."

Using "Bad" Carbs in Interval and Race Strategies

Some like to divide carbs into "good" carbs and "bad" carbs. DeVore prefers "complex" nutrient-dense carbs versus "simple" carbs, which can be understood easily by comparing an orange to orange juice. The former is loaded with fiber; the latter is mostly sugar (fructose), so it results in a much higher insulin spike, which in the long run negatively impacts health. Veggies are carbs that don't spike insulin, which sugar and pasta do, hindering fat utilization, causing inflammation, and raising LDL cholesterol and blood sugar, among with other negative effects.

But as with Zabriskie's pre–weight-lifting diet, "bad" carbs still can help a paleo athlete in intense efforts like intervals and ultradistance races.

Ultrarunners Bitter and Olson both used sugars strategically during their events to give them a boost without upsetting their fat-burning machinery. Olson popped one GU every 4 hours, instead of his previous one per hour, and Bitter downed occasional banana chips in coconut oil, a couple handfuls of potato chips (for the salt), a bag of M&Ms, and some Gatorade and Mountain Dew.

Triathlete Inkinen avoided "bad" carbs (fast-burning sugars and processed-grain foods like orange juice and bagels) at all times except before and after high-intensity interval sessions, which tend to burn and rapidly deplete blood sugar and muscle glycogen. Otherwise, he stuck to a high-fat/moderate-protein/low-carbohydrate diet, featuring eggs, grass-fed beef, butter, nuts, fish, coconut oil, leafy vegetables, some fruits, and dark chocolate. Rojnik had a similar experience, finding that going full-blown "ketogenic"—an extreme paleo state that virtually eliminates carbs—was unsustainable. To stop his carb cravings, thirst, and bad mood, he went back to his low-carb diet but uses gels and sugar in races and carbo-loads the day before a race.

For a healthy life and optimal endurance performance, we believe a paleo diet that turns you into a fat-burning beast is the way to go. It may be that high-intensity intervals and extra-long efforts like ultrarunning or Ironman races appear to require some targeted "bad" carbs, a strategy that may apply to your Maximum Overload workouts as well. Ultimately, you have to experiment and find what is right for your body.

In conclusion, we hope to leave you with two realizations about food and training:

1. Eating fat does not make you fat and unhealthy; eating too much sugar and refined carbs does because they prompt your body to store fat, not burn it.

2. Eating more fat and less carbs makes you faster because you weigh less, get sick less, recover faster,

and develop a fat-burning engine with access to a huge fuel tank (your body fat) that lets you go farther without slowing down.

THE RISE AND FALL OF THE CARBO PARTY

Remember the Carbo Party? The night before the race when you mainlined pasta, pizza, French bread, and cinnamon-raisin donuts?

Suddenly, it's uncool. Younger athletes might not even know what it is, or was. That's because we know now that eating lots of processed carbs isn't good for you. The party's over.

A little history will explain how we got from there to here.

After a half-million years of eating a high-fat/high-protein/natural carb diet, humans domesticated formerly inedible wheat and corn and invented farming 10,000 years ago. We thrived on bread and tortillas. Weaned on an erratic hunter-gatherer fat-protein diet, we blossomed with a constant food supply, even if it was based on foods that were not being eaten in their natural form. Able to sit and think and tend their crops, our ancestors invented the wheel, Broadway plays, and kindergarten. World population exploded, even though we were eating refined grains, the stuff we've been saying for several pages is bad for you. The medical catastrophes of modern life—obesity, diabetes, heart disease—were rare, probably because humans didn't overeat as much as today, still consumed lots of fat and protein, and still had to move around quite a bit.

Then, about 40 years ago, the number of people with

those diseases began to explode. That's because the percentage of carbs and sugar in our diets suddenly surged, the computer workstation became an immobile jail, and "fat" became a dirty word. "High-carb/low-fat" was made a government-mandated policy; heavily processed, unnatural food became the norm; and good-tasting fat was removed from foods and replaced with sweeteners, sending caloric intake and obesity rates through the roof.

Processed, highly profitable foods arose from the lab, such as high fructose corn syrup (HFCS), a laboratory-altered glucose-fructose hybrid processed from cornstarch that was invented by a team of Americans in 1957 and perfected by a Japanese government scientist around 1970. Maybe the single worst food creation of all time, HFCS got a boost from Earl Butz, secretary of agriculture from 1971 to 1976 during the inflation-paranoid Nixon and Ford administrations, who were determined to bring food prices down.

To cut prices, Butz cut the subsidies farmers had long received to *not* grow too much wheat and corn and used tax incentives to prod them to plant their fields "fence post to fence post." He implored them to "get big or get out"—in other words, to consolidate and grow more, which would and did keep prices down. So began large-scale "industrialized farming" and huge grain surpluses, which by the early 1980s were being addressed with novel ideas: feeding corn to cows and the widespread adoption of a new sweetening agent called HFCS.

A third cheaper than sugar and 25 percent sweeter (87 versus 70 on the glycemic index), HFCS flowed directly into the bloodstream of America starting in 1984, when Coke and Pepsi first used it as a sugar replacement. Soon, HFCS was infiltrating everything: ketchup, breakfast cereals, steak sauce, and energy bars. The problem with HFCS, unlike the natural (and relatively minimal at GI 17) fructose in fruit, is that it is so concentrated. Not bound to fiber, it processes through the body faster and leaves you fatter yet unsatiated. That's because HFCS actually encourages overeating and overdrinking by suppressing leptin, a hormone made by fat cells that is supposed to curtail eating by signaling the brain that the fat cells have had enough. Without the leptin stop sign, consumption of soft drinks, already the biggest source of calories of any single food category in the US diet, rose from 350 cans a year to 600 in a decade. Rats fed HFCS gained 40 percent more weight than rats fed the same amount of sugar. By 1994, the Centers for Disease Control and Prevention noted an alarming increase in obesity.

Unfortunately, you're not free of food addiction if you replace your ubiquitous HFCS-laden foods with clones sweetened with old-fashioned sugar, such as the increasingly popular Mexican Coke, imported from south of the border. For years, experts like former FDA commissioner Dr. David Kessler (1990 to 1997) believed that sugar gives you a "hedonic rush" that is wired to the pleasure centers of your brain, creating an addictive-like desire to keep consuming it. This was confirmed in a study published in the December 2013 issue of the *American Journal of Clinical Nutrition*, which found that sugar, more than fat, fuels overeating because it causes greater activation of the gustatory region—the part of the brain responsible for the perception of taste.

Since starches and grains have higher glycemic indexes

than sugar and are also addictive, they are doubly dangerous because they are now found in virtually every food product. On top of that, the overproduction and genetic manipulation of wheat has raised the general exposure to gluten, a protein not tolerated by 15 percent of the population and is linked to fatigue, inflammation, mood swings, and many diseases, allergies, and digestive problems.

Grain-mania isn't the only factor that took us away from healthy primal eating. The deification of carbs merged with an earlier demonization of fat in the 1950s that was set in motion by the influential researcher Ancel Keys, the inventor of K-rations, a 3,200-calorie, ready-to-eat meal-in-a-box for World War II soldiers. Keys had no intrinsic dislike of fat, but his studies of heart-attack–prone Minnesota businessmen and amazingly healthy centenarians in southern Italy led him to conclude that animal fats caused the high serum cholesterol associated with coronary heart disease.

There was only one problem with that analysis: It was wrong. Animal fats aren't only not bad for you, but they're actually good for you. It took 50 years to fix that mistake.

When Keys, who would later be celebrated on the January 13, 1961, cover of *Time* magazine as a diet guru, said "go low-fat," the government paid attention. (Keys practiced what he preached, by the way, as he spent the last 28 years of his life eating a low-fat diet on the southwest coast of Italy, before dying at age 100 in 2004.) His conclusion that saturated fats from milk and meat were harmful and that unsaturated fats from vegetable oils were beneficial led to a 1956 nationwide TV appearance by representatives of the American Heart Association. Their message: Eating large amounts of butter, lard, eggs, and beef would lead to coronary heart disease.

So, "low-fat" became the law of the land. Margarine makers were thrilled. Generations of kids grew up on gallons of watery 2 percent fat milk. Low-fat diet books sold in the millions. So entrenched was the low-fat orthodoxy that no one questioned it for decades, until someone began to notice something weird:

We're eating and drinking low-fat everything, **but we're getting more and more messed up.** We're fatter and more diabetic by the hour. What's going on?

The first major attempt to answer that question came in the 1972 book *Pure, White, and Deadly* by British physiologist and nutritionist John Yudkin. It cited evidence that the over-consumption of sugar was the main cause of heart disease and a key player in diabetes, cancer, and other diseases. The sugar industry and Keys, who had given sugar a free pass in his studies, fought back and discredited Yudkin. However, in the years after his death in 1995, Yudkin would ultimately emerge a hero when his findings were confirmed.

Actually, the first major crack in the anti-fat wall came in a 1992 editorial published in the *Archives of Internal Medicine* by Dr. William Castelli, a former director of the Framingham Heart Study, which began tracking the diet and lifestyle habits of 6,000 people in Framingham, Massachusetts in 1948. The study identified heart-disease risk factors, such as smoking, high blood pressure, lack of exercise, and high cholesterol, but did not blame dietary saturated fat. "In Framingham, we found that the people who ate the most saturated fat and the most cholesterol had the lower serum cholesterol," Dr. Castelli said. "(That was) the opposite of what . . . Keys et al. would predict."

Over time, more studies began to blame heart problems and the exploding diabetes rate on sugar, refined carbohydrates, and the unsaturated fats in vegetable oils instead of the saturated fats in meat. In 2008, Gary Taubes' bestseller *Good Calories, Bad Calories* stood the Keys anti-saturated fat orthodoxy on its head by showing that low-cholesterol diets had almost no effect on blood-cholesterol levels and that low-fat diets had a minimal effect on life span. His follow-up books, *Why We Get Fat* and *The Case Against Sugar*, gave more fuel to the growing paleo movement.

When last decade saw a flood of natural-food diet plans and books hit the market, including Sisson's *Primal Blueprint*, success stories sprang up by the thousands—and fat haters had to start changing their tunes. Even a died-in-the-wool low-fat warrior like Dr. Mehmet Oz.

On April 17, 2014, the famed TV doctor shocked millions by saying, "I was wrong about dietary fat.

"It is turning out that saturated fat—the stuff we thought was bad for you—is actually good for you," he said. "It's healthy. And it turns out that the stuff we thought was good for you—processed grains—is actually bad for you." Grains caused inflammation, spiked insulin, and caused heart disease, diabetes . . . the list was endless. So Dr. Oz went paleo.

Dr. Oz reversed his position in light of overwhelming scientific evidence, particularly an October 2013 declaration by esteemed British cardiologist Aseem Malhotra showing that a high-fat, low-carb diet featuring unprocessed saturated fat actually has a protective effect against heart disease, diabetes, and dementia. Saturated fat was actually the body's preferred fuel. In fact, Dr. Oz had already aired a show with neurologist David Perlmutter, who said a heavily saturated fat diet could prevent and even reverse Alzheimer's.

So the point was irrefutably made in front of America and the world: The fat-is-evil maxim of the last 50 years was dead wrong. The great Oz said so! Good fat is actually good for you. Bad carbs—sugar and processed carbs—are bad for you.

Ancel Keys was surely retching in his grave. How could he have been so wrong? According to Nina Teicholz, author of the 2014 bestseller *The Big Fat Surprise: Why Butter, Meat and Cheese Belong in a Healthy Diet*, Keys was guilty of editing his research. "He undercounted the saturated fats [his study subject ate and] missed entirely that they ate no sugar and vegetable oils," Teicholz wrote. "He focused on what he wanted to see."[1]

Time magazine's June 22, 2014, issue settled the debate once and for all. Over a dramatic photo of a piece of bright yellow butter set against a black background, the stark headline on the cover read, "Eat Butter." The subhead read, "Scientists labeled fat the enemy. Why they were wrong." The eight-page story presented some of the same research exonerating dietary fat that was cited here and pointed to the "overconsumption of carbohydrates, sugar, and sweeteners that is chiefly responsible for the epidemics of obesity and Type 2 diabetes." The true villains, according to *Time*: bread, pasta, and crackers, which encourage the body to store calories as fat and intensify hunger, making it difficult to lose weight.

Unfortunately, the US government moves slowly. The 2015–2020 dietary recommendations didn't back-off on its 30-year-old anti-fat message, although it does say to eat less sugar. In doing so, the government did not listen to a radical rewriting of the rules pushed by its own Dietary Guidelines Advisory Committee (DGAC), a panel of scientists who advise the secretaries of Agriculture and Health and Human Services. DGAC's 2015 report was radical because its recommendations reversed nearly 4 decades of anti-saturated fat nutrition policy: Eat all the saturated fat you want (as there was no evidence that it raised heart-disease risk or caused obesity), cut bad fats such as trans-fats, and generally stick to "healthful diet patterns that include more vegetables, fruits, whole grains, seafood, legumes, and dairy products and include less meat, sugar-sweetened foods and drinks, and refined grains."[2]

The bottom line: The half-century–long disinformation campaign is over. It is refined carbs and man-made vegetable oils that are bad for you, not fat. When cultural bellwethers like *Time* magazine and Dr. Oz finally get religion, society pays attention and millions reap the benefits, including endurance athletes. In fact, it turns out that the longer you go, the more the benefits, which is why long-distance riders, runners, rowers, and triathletes may have more to gain from low-carb/high-fat than any other athletes. Their sustained aerobic pace can keep them solidly in fat-burning mode for many hours.

Diet, the new performance-enhancing drug?

FINAL WORD: WHY WEIGHTS ARE TOO GOOD TO PASS UP

Healthy muscles. Beautiful bones. Better, longer quality of life. And—oh yeah—you'll go faster on a bike.

Jacques DeVore doesn't expect everyone to love Maximum Overload. He acknowledges that the conversation is just beginning, and he knows his baby will be tweaked and rejiggered and rejected. "But after looking at all the evidence," he says, "I'd be shocked if anyone doubts the broader topic of weight training for cyclists. Because it's a must."

Weight training is a must for improving your cycling performance—and there is a growing body of academic studies to prove it, which you'll see in a minute. But more important, heavy weight training, like that advocated in

Maximum Overload, is a must for your quality of life—for two reasons: It protects muscles. It protects bones. Protect them both, and you end up with greatly enhanced health, fitness, and longevity.

Both muscles and bones naturally begin an alarming life-long deterioration starting in your 30s, and cycling does not stop it. In fact, in the case of bones, cyclists who ride a bike only for fitness actually can accelerate the deterioration, literally forcing their skeletons into osteoporosis. This is not a rare occurrence. If you ride a lot, are over 40, and don't do any serious gravity and/or impact activities like running, backpacking, or weight lifting, you most likely already have some degree of accelerated bone thinning.

Scared yet? We hope so. Maybe that'll get you lifting weights—even if you don't necessarily have a burning desire to stand on the podium.

We'll discuss the positive impact of weight training on maintaining cyclists' bone and muscle mass later in this chapter. First, we'll wrap up the discussion of why weights in general are good for performance by citing research that supports DeVore's success stories with Dave Zabriskie, Denise Mueller, and many local amateur racers (see the sidebars on some of them in Chapters 2, 4, and 6). A small but growing body of academic studies has found that weight training indeed makes cyclists faster. By overloading your muscles in the weight room far more than you can by riding outdoors, researchers discovered that weights can develop a superior type and quantity of muscle fibers that fatigue later in the race, protect you against injuries that interrupt your training, and ultimately give you the vaunted Maximum Sustainable

Power (MSP)—the key to holding form and speed throughout the race and having enough left for a strong finish.

Studies published in international sports-medicine journals not only support DeVore and other pro-weights advocates, but also show that test groups made gains from surprisingly simple additions to their normal on-the-road cycling training programs—with routines nowhere near as complex as Maximum Overload. The test riders typically did limited, surprisingly simple weight-lifting exercises: half-squats, single-leg presses, or leg extensions several times a week for a month or two. Yet they yielded very positive results for cyclists of all ages, with substantial benefits often accruing to masters riders. DeVore notes that relatively small improvement in power adds up over a bike race, with a 1 percent differential in a 40-kilometer time trial often cutting 45 seconds.

A 2014 meta-analysis, a summary of previous studies (see below), concluded that heavy weight training could lead to significant increases in power, economy, and performance for cyclists. This does not come from adding lots of new muscle mass (which would have negative implications for the power-to-weight ratio so important in cycling). The gains are neurological, which means that they have to come from strengthening your existing muscle fibers, both the endurance-oriented slow-twitch type and the speed- and power-oriented fast-twitch type.

For example: Researchers found that use of heavy weights strengthened and increased the time it takes to exhaust slow-twitch muscle fibers, thereby reserving your fast-twitch fibers for later in the race. Others discovered that heavy weight training is better than light, high-rep training for building powerful "high performance" type IIA fast-twitch muscle fibers that don't exhaust as easily as the type IIAX to IIX fibers they replace. When your rivals are exhausted on the last couple hill climbs, type IIAs are the ones that can give you that final oomph you need to pass them.

Here's a small sample of those studies and other recent research:

- **2016:** Heavy strength training with one-leg leg presses made well-trained female cyclists faster in a 40-minute time trial, due to increased quadriceps strength and an upgrade of fast-twitch muscle fibers from type IIAX to IIX to higher-performance type IIA.[1]

- **2014:** A meta-study found that adding strength training to an endurance athlete's program causes improved economy, muscle power, and performance. (But it wasn't sure about what exercises, mix of exercises, training intensities, and duration of program were best.)[2]

- **2013:** In this study of runners and cyclists, researchers found "compelling" evidence of increased cycling endurance performance with heavy strength training, possibly due to delayed activation of less efficient type II fibers, improved neuromuscular efficiency, conversion of fast-twitch type IIX fibers into more fatigue-resistant type IIA fibers, or improved musculotendinous stiffness.[3]

- **2012:** Masters cyclists saw significant improvement in muscle performance from a 3-week program of knee-extension exercises—much more pronounced than the effect on younger cyclists.[4]

- **2011:** Heavy weight training helped young, elite competitive cyclists improve 45-minute time-trial times more than light, high-rep training. This correlated to an increased proportion of type IIA muscle fibers relative to more easily exhausted type IIX muscle fibers, and gains in muscle strength and power.[5]

- **2010:** Eight weeks of half-squats improved cycling economy and time to exhaustion in competitive cyclists—and even more in untrained cyclists.[6]

- **2010:** A survey of published studies concluded that it is likely that replacing a portion of a cyclist's endurance training with resistance training (including high-intensity explosive exercises) will result in improved time-trial performance and maximal power.[7]

The upshot of all this is clear: It is not DeVore's wishful thinking that weight training can increase a cyclist's strength, endurance, power production, and resilience to injury. Without necessarily adding bulk and large amounts of muscle fiber, a wide range of studies confirms that weight training allows you to use your existing muscle more efficiently, tap into formerly unused power, and perform better late in your races and events.

As mentioned before, keep in mind that while the research experiments listed above generally use heavy weights to elicit the greatest response, those studies are often limited to isolated muscles or exercises. Lacking thus far is a comprehensive study of heavy weight lifting and it's impact on a maximum sustainable power program like Maximum Overload that hits a variety of muscles. That kind of complexity might make it difficult to isolate cause and effect in a study.

But think about it: If significant benefits can come out of merely hitting the quadriceps with leg extensions (the 2012 study) or doing four sets of four half-squats three times a week (the 2010 study), imagine the gains from a full-bore 40- to 60-minute workout that includes deadlifts, Bulgarian split squats, walking lunges, lat pulls, and core exercises.

After all, cycling involves far more than quads and legs. In the three phases that make up the motion of cycling (downstroke, upstroke, and pushing to reach top dead center of the crank cycle), a rider uses the gluteus maximus, hamstrings, calves, and anterior shin muscles (tibialis anterior) as well as the mighty quads. In addition, upper-body and core muscles play a key role in stabilizing the bike and creating a solid foundation that the legs can leverage off of for power. That's why DeVore designed the Maximum Overload program to activate, straighten, and strengthen the core, back, and shoulders before moving on to the complex, multijoint exercises that blast the mover muscles of the legs and hips in an attempt to develop MSP.

Of course, coaches and athletes in other sports—football, basketball, baseball, soccer, skiing, you name it—have known for decades that stronger muscles are more "efficient," which means that they can do more work with the same effort. That was confirmed academically back in 1994 in a study that identified changes to muscle-fiber activation patterns in before-and-after MRIs of quadriceps worked out twice a week for 2 months.[8] But the benefit to endurance athletes, especially cyclists and runners, remained unknown and ignored.

That will change as so-called concurrent training (the official term for workout programs that mix endurance and weight workouts) is studied more and programs like Maximum Overload successfully train more cyclists. As the word gets out, DeVore is convinced that weight training and MSP training will soon be not only the norm in cycling, but also become an absolute necessity for those who aspire to the podium—as common to cycling training plans as intervals and tempo rides.

It'll also use up less time. The aforementioned 2010 study shows that replacing a road workout with a gym workout yields better results than piling a weight workout on top of your regular riding schedule. Future serious cyclists—from pros to club riders—will actually spend less cumulative time working out. Here's why.

The improvement in strength and power you get from weight training builds upon itself. It's like "the rich get richer." You get more overloads in every workout you do—sprints, tempo workouts, time trialing, hill climbing, and track workouts. If you used to reach the mailbox in your old hill repeats and now can go two houses farther, that workout now makes you fitter than it did before. All your hours on the bike have greater value to you—which is why you can get away with doing less of them under the Maximum Overload program.

Speaking of time, weight training can be like turning back the clock. The primary difference between the 18-year-old cyclist and the masters cyclist is that the youngster

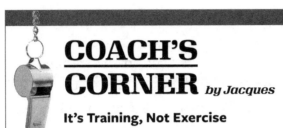

COACH'S
CORNER *by Jacques*

It's Training, Not Exercise

I say it all the time: "It's training, not exercise"—a mantra I repeat to my staff and my clients continually. Those words are the reason why I got into this business, and why people from pro athletes to 68-year-old grandmas seek out my services. Because training and exercise are not the same thing.

I want to train people—for performance and for life. I want to make them better—now, a year from now, and a decade from now. You want mere exercise? Go to a Group-X class at your local gym and jump up and down for 50 minutes. Work up a good sweat. But do you want to learn a system that'll make you faster, fitter, better—and teach you how to stay that way long after you stop paying me? That's training—and that's what I always wanted to do, starting with myself and my friends nearly two decades ago.

Maximum Overload is the end result of all my years of tinkering and strategizing about training, of objectively evaluating the body's strengths and weaknesses, and of assessing progress from one point in time to another. It came about because I dared to ask the question "why?" Why, I wondered, are we just doing what has been done in the past? Why do people in the gym do three sets of 10? Why do cyclists train only one dimension of power and not Maximum Sustainable Power (MSP)? Why do cyclists today train the same way cyclists did 30 years ago—and never touch a weight? Why do aerobic athletes only do aerobic training? Why do athletes add strength but ignore power, the thing that they really need to win the race?

Because they don't ask why.

Knowledge gets passed down from generation to generation—

recovers fasters and produces greater power and bigger over-loads while the oldster sees diminishing power and overloads. The mailbox is getting farther and farther away from him. But

but how sensible and effective is that knowledge to start with? The "why" is oftentimes never really understood, so I insist that my coaches and clients understand the "why."

Maximum Overload is a work in progress that I'm hoping will spur knockoffs and improvements. But I think its big idea—that weight training is essential for building an endurance athlete's MSP—is undeniable. Here's why:

Endurance athletes, and particularly cyclists, require a high power-to-weight ratio. Most endurance coaches focus on the aerobic engine and how to sustain the highest percentage of an athlete's VO_2 max (absolute aerobic power) for the longest period of time. Little attention is spent on how to produce more sustainable power in the muscles, particularly the legs. If you can train your legs to produce greater amounts of power over long periods of time, you don't deteriorate as fast. That, in a nutshell, is the goal of the Maximum Overload program.

Again, why look only at aerobic power? Why not see if our bodies with proper training design will be able to produce greater and greater amounts of power? Could you train less? Could you be a better version of your current highly fit self? Could you take power outputs to a level you never thought possible? This book, the Maximum Overload philosophy, and the relentless pursuit of MSP are based on these "whys."

Ultimately, there's no compelling reason to ask why if all you want is exercise. Just lace up your shoes and go for a run or do a boot camp. But if you want to be a better bike racer, a better masters athlete, or a fitter, more functional, more robust grandparent who lives life to the fullest while your peers are locking themselves in prisons of inactivity, you must be trained. Maximum Overload is your training.

with a small amount of the time in the weight room, he or she can bring that power and bigger overloads back, maybe reach the mailbox again, and close the gap with the youngster.

SAVING MUSCLE AND BONE

Although performance was the subject of the aforementioned academic studies, the enhanced safety and functionality of strength training repeatedly come up in them. From the 2012 study: "In masters, the strength training induced an enhancement in maximal and endurance torque production and cycling efficiency, thus reducing age-related differences in performance recorded before training. These results suggest that strength training added to endurance training might be a complementary strategy to preserve functional capacity and performance with aging."

Functional capacity means good posture, strength, quickness, full range of motion, and being able to do the same things you like doing now 30 years from now, all of which require healthy muscles and bones.

Muscles are life. Bones are life. Robust, youthful ones make you strong, mobile, flexible, and functional. Unfortunately and surprisingly, aging—and cycling!—are not kind to muscles and bones. Many old cyclists in their 70s (actually, there aren't many of them, for this reason) have frail, hesitantly moving, stooped-over, bag-of-bones bodies that seem almost devoid of muscular power and skeletal integrity, as if they are vaporizing into dust. Well, sadly, they are. But it doesn't have to be. There is no reason why you shouldn't continue to be a monster on the bike—and off of it—into your 70s and 80s.

This section discusses the nasty one-two punch that aging and cycling inflict on cyclists' muscles and bones—and what you can do about it. Not surprisingly, the number-one solution on the list is what these last few pages have been talking about: weight training.

How to Maintain Muscle Mass

Muscles grow larger and stronger until some point in your 30s, when size and function (and related strength and mobility) start to decline, a condition known as age-related sarcopenia, which can cause muscle-mass declines of 3 percent to 10 percent per decade (depending on which article you read) into your 70s, when the loss accelerates. The root causes of sarcopenia are aging, inactivity, and an incomplete diet, which together lead to several interrelated problems: reduction of the nerve cells that send signals to move from the brain to the muscles; a decrease in quantity of muscle-building hormones such as testosterone, HGH, and insulin-like growth factor; and a decrease in the supply of protein and the ability to synthesize it.

There's one more cause of sarcopenia, which might seem counterintuitive: a catabolic (muscle breakdown) effect of endurance training. Long bouts of moderate-paced, low-intensity aerobics like cycling and long-distance running can outrun their supply of glycogen fuel, forcing a release of hormones such as cortisol that work to break down muscle tissue.

That's the bad news. The good news is that you can fight back immediately, slowing the pace of muscle-mass deterioration and even reversing it with the right activity and fuel. Unfortunately, cycling alone is not the right activity.

Although you'd hope that cycling's rigorous hill climbing

and hard efforts would create enough overload to force your body to build muscle faster than aging can break it down, that is not the case. Most "hard" riding is simply not hard enough to set off the body's alarm bells. Upper-body muscles, which get minimal work on a bike no matter how hard you ride, will continue to shrivel by the standard 1-plus percent a year. As for the lower body, the muscle-mass decline in the legs can be slowed but not stopped for all but track riders, whose repeated hard sprint efforts can approach the overload of a weight workout. Sprints, as discussed in Chapter 6, are the aerobic counterpart of heavy, high-performance weight training.

By now, you can probably write much of the next paragraph yourself: If you want to stop age-related muscle-mass decline and resuscitate your withered sinew, you need the high, concentrated levels of overload and adaptation of what you get from heavy weight lifting and intervals. Going to failure and near-failure levels leaves in their wake microtears in the proteins that control the muscles' contraction. These temporarily damaged muscles send a message to the brain that they need some extra protein to heal the tears and rebuild themselves even stronger in order to withstand another assault. An army of anabolic (muscle-building) hormones, including testosterone (T), a performance-enhancer that aids postexercise recovery, and human growth hormone (HGH), the body's antiaging fountain of youth, is dispatched from the pituitary gland. Note that T, already undergoing a long natural decline with age and further diminished during bouts of lengthy, cortisol-releasing aerobic exercise, will see a huge spurt in production during activities of great intensity and overload, such as heavy weight training and intervals. (Dietary fat also boosts T, making fat a smart recovery fuel.) Likewise, the body's HGH production after 40 or 50, which has slumped to a fraction of the amount once used to grow you from a kid into an adult, temporarily surges back with the hard efforts of weights and sprints. HGH helps glue your torn muscles back together; grow your muscle mass; improve bone, cartilage, hair, nails, and skin; stimulate deeper sleep; and even reduce body fat.

The bottom line: If you're a cyclist over 40, long-term health demands that you hit the gym hard a couple times a week, do an interval session, and eat more protein, the building blocks of muscle. Before you know it, those age-withered muscles will quickly regain some of their pretty, long-ago plumpness and the youthful vigor that come along with them.

How to Maintain Bone Density

Withered muscles are one thing. They look bad, reduce your function, lower your performance potential, and provide less metabolic protection against illnesses and traumatic injuries, but at least they respond very quickly to workouts and can be rebuilt. Within a few weeks of training, you can see and feel muscular improvements. But your skeleton is another story.

When your bones get hollow and thin, it makes you subject to catastrophic failure that can put you out of commission for weeks or months—or life. You might expect age-withered bones to come along with withered muscles, right? But what if we told you that your well-toned biker-built leg muscles are hiding wimpy, hollowed-out bones—and that cycling was actually causing the hollowing?

And what if you found out that anyone who only rides a bike and does no cross-training or weight training is probably on the road to osteoporosis?

Fact: If all you do is ride, you're a broken hip waiting to happen. You probably already have significant bone thinning. To stop it and reverse it, you must lift weights.

"Anyone who rides a bike as his or her main form of fitness is risking osteoporosis," says Jeanne Nichols, a masters racer and exercise-physiology professor at California State University at San Diego, who established the cycling–bone loss connection with a landmark bone-density study of cyclists published in 2003.[9] Described that year in a *Bicycling* magazine article entitled "Why You Need to Bone Up,"[10] by *Maximum Overload for Cyclists* coauthor Roy Wallack, the study used DXA machines to measure the bone densities of 26 male masters cyclists, who had trained an average of 12.2 hours per week for 20 years. The eye-opening results: Two-thirds of the test group had osteopenia—noticeable bone thinning. Four had full-blown osteoporosis—severe thinning. All this at an average age of 51, when most normal men have no bone thinning at all.

Nichols' research and the *Bicycling* article led to hundreds of similar articles and research studies into the topic over the next decade, and the conclusions were all the same: The unique non-weight-bearing, nonimpact nature of cycling, in which your body weight is supported by a bike seat, demotivates the body to maintain your skeleton. Cyclists' bones are subject to much less stress than those of athletes whose skeletons support their own weight against gravity on land—like runners, soccer players, and cross-country skiers. In terms of bone stress, cyclists are more like astronauts living in the International Space Station (who always return with severely wasted skeletons): Every moment their feet don't touch the Earth, calcium is draining away. (Calcium loss through sweat is another key factor, as you'll see later.)

Typical of Nichols' study group was Bill Holland, a well-known San Diego custom bike builder. Age 48 at the time of Nichols' study, the 5-foot-10, 147-pound rider told Wallack that he was superfit and looked 10 years younger than his age. He had been riding 150 miles a week for 25 years. So when the results of his DXA scans showed he had borderline osteoporosis, he was shocked.

"A doctor told me that I had the heart and lungs of a 17-year-old," says Holland, "and the bones of a 70-year-old."

He confirmed that diagnosis a few weeks later with a 15-mph crash that left him with a fractured left hip, broken collarbone, and a bunch of cracked ribs. "At that (slow) speed, my riding buddies didn't think anyone's bones could break, but I couldn't get up," he said.

The idea that athletic men with superfit hearts, lungs, and legs could have the brittle skeletons of doddering grannies was shocking, especially since osteoporosis affects women far more than men. But after digesting the news, cyclists thought it made sense. No wonder we break our collarbones so much!

The osteoporosis-cycling linkage was unknown to the public and to most researchers, though several studies had preceded Nichols', such as a 1996 report on four Tour de

France riders that showed a mean loss of about 25 percent of their spinal bone mass over the course of the race.[11] Dozens of studies have followed Nichols', with similar findings, some even saying, for bone health, it's better to do nothing than ride a bike. "In spite of the elevated muscle contractions inherent to the activity," said a 2010 report that compared 30 young pro riders to same-aged nonathletes, the pros showed "significant bone thinning" throughout their skeletons—especially the femur (–18 percent at the neck of the thigh bone).[12] A 2008 study of 14 male cyclists showed that BMD decreased significantly at the total hip, neck, trochanter, and shaft regions.[13] The studies don't all agree; the last one did not show bone deterioration at the lumbar spine, while others show cyclists' lumbar spine at greatest risk. Any way you look at it, the overall news is bad for lots of riding and bone loss.

A 7-year study of male masters riders published in 2011 found that nearly 90 percent of the subjects had osteoporosis or osteopenia, a far higher rate than the noncyclist control group.[14]

What was the solution, beyond riding less? The authors of the latter study recommended this: "Coaches and health professionals interacting with cyclists need to promote alternative exercise such as weight training, plyometrics, or other high impact activity as a complement to cycle training to help minimize bone loss in this population."

There it is again: **weight training!**

To cue the body to build bone, cyclists need to add load-bearing activities like running, jumping, and lifting weights. And if you must ride, try off-road, where you'll get some jarring; a 2002 study found that mountain bikers had denser bones than roadies.[15]

Making things worse for cyclists is a double-whammy Nichols and other researchers hadn't considered: Cyclists lose a ton of calcium through sweat.

A 2-year study of college basketball players beginning in the 1994–95 season at the University of Memphis, led by Robert Klesges, found significant bone loss during the 6-month season and summer practices.[16] He and his researchers discovered why after practice when they wrung out the players' jerseys and analyzed the sweat. Klesges said he found "huge expenditures of sodium, which we expected, and surprising amounts of calcium, which we didn't."

It turns out that an average-size man can sweat out up to 200 milligrams of calcium in an hour of vigorous exercise, according to Christine Snow of the Oregon State University Bone Research Laboratory. "That shouldn't be a problem for average people," she said. But when reminded that cyclists sometimes ride all day, the math became frightening. At an average of 12.2 hours a week, Nichols' test subjects lost over 2,400 milligrams of calcium—2 days' worth of their USRDA per week for years. No wonder their bones were wasting away.

To some extent, what comes out can be put back in. During the next basketball season at Memphis, Klesges stirred 2,000 milligrams of low-cost calcium lactate into each player's energy drinks. The results of the supplementation: In the 1995–96 season, "bone loss was virtually eliminated," said Klesges. For the next 5 years, Memphis players continued to drink extra calcium, with the same results.

(continued on page 230)

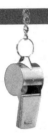

COAUTHOR'S
CORNER *by Roy*

Maximum Overload's 147-mph Woman

On September 12, 2016, on Utah's Bonneville Salt Flats, Denise Mueller set a world record by riding a bike 147.7 mph. Yes: 1- 4 -7. Twice the interstate highway speed limit and about two-and-a-half times the original record of the legendary Charles "Mile-a-Minute" Murphy, who in 1899 set the first paced bicycle speed record of 1 mile in 57.8 seconds behind a motor vehicle (in his case, a train). Denise, drafting 3 feet behind a modified Range Rover SVR as it punched a hole in the air, is now listed as the world's fastest female cyclist in the *Guinness Book of World Records* and—in the eyes of the appreciative authors of this book—is the premier poster child for Maximum Overload.

How big a role did Maximum Overload play in Denise's record? After all, she'd done the MO workouts as much as three times a week from January through September 2016, building up to an impressive 230-pound deadlift. She was quick to give MO inventor Jacques DeVore credit as her power output rose (both on the walking-lunge MSP tests and on the bike) and her race victories piled up over the spring and summer. So at Bonneville, did Maximum Overload make Mueller 1 mph faster? 5 mph faster? 10 mph faster?

Asked to give an estimate, Mueller and her coach John Howard both settled on 5 mph—with a caveat: It could have been double or triple that. Trouble was, they got rained out.

They knew for a fact that Maximum Overload had had a huge effect on her power—up a whopping 20 percent, which allowed her to hold a sustained surge of 800-plus watts. Unfortunately, a rain-shortened course limited her chance to get up to a speed that would require her full power; the data showed that 147.7 mph was easy for Mueller, pushing her to just over 700 watts. It is in the harder effort range from 700 to 800 watts that Maximum Overload would really pay off. In other words, MO worked, but Mueller had a lot more gas in the tank. (*Note:* Mueller's MO-augmented power in an all-out, finish-line sprint was much higher, around 1,260 watts.)

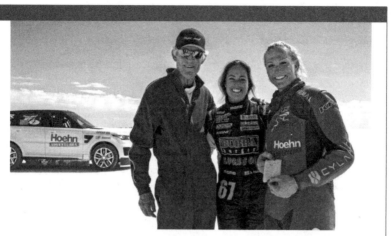

Coach John Howard, driver Shea Holbrook, and Denise Mueller celebrate her 147.7 mph run.

So even at 147.7 mph, Mueller hadn't scratched the surface of her Maximum Overload–bred power potential. Here's the backstory.

Mueller, once a teenage champion, does everything all out, and Maximum Overload, a late addition to her Bonneville training, was no exception. That she did the program at all was due to her open-minded coach, Howard, who set a record of 152.2 mph in 1985.

In January 2016, seeking more Maximum Overload case studies for the book alongside Dave Zabriskie and a few amateur racers, I called Howard. I'd interviewed the three-time Olympian and Cycling Hall of Fame member many times over the years and featured him in my book *Bike for Life: How to Ride to 100*. I'd always admired his curiosity and creativity, his willingness to push the envelope in the Hawaii Ironman triathlon, the Race Across America (RAAM) and the speed record, and try new training ideas. So now I made the pitch.

"John, we're writing a book about a radical new cycling training program that flies in the face of 100 years of conventional cycling wisdom. It's the first one that claims to increase sustainable power with something no cycling coach in his right mind would ever recommend: heavy weight lifting.

"I'm looking for a high-profile guinea pig to try it on. Ideally, someone older, still competitive, who desperately wants to maintain or even raise his power, and has the creativity, confidence, and sheer balls

(continues)

Maximum Overload's 147-mph Woman (*cont.*)

enough to experiment with something that would scare the average rider away. The only one I know of who fits that description is you."

I told Howard how MO had worked for Zabriskie and explained Jacques' big idea: that the limiting factor of an endurance athlete was not only aerobic fitness, but also muscular power—which heavy weights can build better than riding itself. He was intrigued. I gave him Jacques' phone number.

A week later, when Howard showed up at Jacques' gym at 6:30 a.m. on a Sunday, he surprised us by bringing along a bubbly, robust 43-year-old with long blonde hair and an addictive enthusiasm. Mueller, a mother of three who ran a home-security business, was a former junior national champion ranked the No. 1 US junior in 1991. She'd racked up 13 national titles in road, track, and mountain bike racing and two podium finishes in the junior world championships, then retired at age 20 in 1993, burned out by the sport and eager to move on to married life. She didn't race again until Howard, who'd coached her as a teen, ran into her by chance in 2012.

Impressed by Mueller's general fitness, he proposed something crazy: that she return to bike racing and attempt what only nine people—and no woman—had ever tried before: the paced land speed record. He was convinced she would not only set an impressive first-time women's record, but was capable of becoming the outright record holder, breaking both his own 1985 record of 152.2 mph and the record that broke his: that of Dutch pro Fred Rompelberg, whom Howard coached to an astounding 167.994 mph in 1995.

Howard and Mueller kept the project secret for 2 years, afraid someone else would steal it. But it turns out that no other woman cared to try.

Ironically, Mueller hadn't been in a bike race for 22 years when Howard ran into her. She'd kept in shape with gym workouts, marathons, and triathlons. Most important for Howard, he felt she still had the drive to do something great in cycling.

We noticed that drive on her first day in the gym.

Instantly, from the start of their first Maximum Overload workout, Mueller easily outlifted the 25-years-older Howard. Her body was balanced and posture straight, like his wasn't. She even followed instructions better than he did. Very strong and powerful, she lifted heavy weights easily, joyously.

Jacques and I looked at each other. We just found our perfect guinea pig for the book.

Over the next 8 months, Mueller drove up for a dozen Sunday-morning workouts at Jacques' gym and religiously did Maximum Overload twice a week at her home gym in Encinitas, e-mailing us meticulous records of her workouts. As her walking-lunge Maximum Sustainable Power (MSP) test numbers in the gym rose, so did her power and results on the bike, including impressive wins against much younger rivals at the Barrio Logan criterium in May and the Carlsbad Grand Prix in July. She was very quick to credit Maximum Overload for her fresh legs in final sprints of those events. "It definitely increases my ability to put out watts and power," she said. Howard agreed.

In September, at the annual Speed Week on the Bonneville Salt Flats in Utah, Howard repeatedly brought up Denise's Maximum Overload–bred power in pre-event interviews. "She's a freak at 43 years old—as strong as she's ever been," he said. "Maybe stronger. She's gained a tremendous amount of raw power. She can deadlift 230 pounds. She can put down 1,300 watts in a snap of finger. That's the kind of power it takes to do this kind of an effort."

Given good salt conditions, Howard was sure Mueller would break his 152.2-mph mark and at least threaten Rompelberg's near-168 mph.

Going that fast in the draft of a speeding car is amazing but can have frightening consequences. On his first record attempt in 1992, Rompelberg wiped out, was knocked unconscious, and took 3 years to recover from his 16 broken bones.

The danger of a wipeout comes from leaving the vortex, the small cocoon of drag-free air behind the vehicle, before slowing down to under 80 to 90 mph; at higher speeds, the friction of the unbroken air outside the fairing-shrouded draft of the vehicle can slam you like a heavyweight punch and make you lose control of the bike.

The big day arrived on September 12. After a few slow-speed runs behind the pace car on her highly engineered single-speed carbon-fiber bike, which featured low-profile 17-inch motorcycle tires, an elongated 27-inch wheelbase for stability, and two giant, 60-tooth

(continues)

Maximum Overload's 147-mph Woman (*cont.*)

chainrings that propelled the bike 130 feet on one crank revolution, Mueller and pro driver Shea Holbrook dialed in their coordination. Pulled to 75, 80, and 85 mph on a tow bar 3 feet behind the $112,000 Range Rover Sport SVR, the world's fastest production SUV, she began pedaling in earnest. That was not possible at lower speeds as the massive gear made it "like starting a car in fifth gear," says Howard.

Wearing a 12-pound leather racing uniform with Kevlar reinforcement at the knees and elbows, Mueller released a spring-loaded line and detached from the pace car at just over 90 mph. She pushed it faster and faster, to 120, 130, 140 mph.

As the speeds rose, the Maximum Overload effect kicked in.

"It gave her the strength that she never had before," said Howard. "Pushing bigger gears—and pushing them explosively—was much easier for her. That explosive power was very valuable in the back-and-forth—an 'oscillation' in the vortex between the rider and the driver that we call 'the Dance.'"

In the Dance, Mueller would bump against the back of the car, bounce back to the back edge of the vortex, then have to push it hard again to catch up to the car. "The surge was very much like the maximum sustainable power test in the gym with the walking lunges," she says. "The push-off in the walking-lunge motion emulated the oscillation."

"Because of her strength," Howard says, "she was able to get back up to the front faster. Because of her strength, Denise was definitely more efficient at choreographing the Dance."

On run number four, Mueller danced her way to 147.7 mph.

They were just getting started. "Shea and I had just cracked the code," Mueller says. "Remember, we'd never done this before. By the fourth run, we figured out the Dance. My surges got smoother as I went faster. We were sure we'd get 155 mph on the fifth run."

Bonneville is 12 miles of dead-flat, 80-foot-wide salt-covered surface. Despite a rain-shortened 4-mile course, a mile less than that used on Howard's and Rompelberg's record runs, Mueller's team was certain they'd hit 155 mph. But pushing past the 167.9 record, they knew, required a 5th mile they didn't have.

Unfortunately, a next-day's fifth run was rained out. The disappointed team had to settle for 147.7 mph, attributing 5 mph of it to Maximum Overload.

"With the short course and limited runs, we ran out of time to take full advantage of my 800-plus watt power," she says. "At 147 mph, I only got to 700-plus sustainable watts on my surges from the back of the vortex. That is, I wasn't close to my limit. Although 20 percent stronger, I couldn't utilize all of it at the lower speeds." She guesses 12 to 14 percent of her power was used.

Guessing the increased mph Mueller gained due to MO is an inexact science. But she and Howard agree it was a key part of her training—certainly the reason for her racing victories earlier in the year, giving her more gas in the tank in the final sprints. Better conditions at Bonneville might have yielded speeds of 155-plus mph, with Maximum Overload possibly contributing 10, 15, even 20 mph of that.

Despite the rain-stunted effort, Mueller drove home happy. "I got to be the first woman to set this record," she said, "and after all, 147 is still pretty fast."

When asked if going double freeway speeds scared her, Mueller would have none of it. "It's exhilarating," she replied. "It's like an amusement park ride. When I'd bump against the bubble, it would shove me forward."

Her anxiety-free reaction to going 147 mph on two wheels may seem eerie to regular folk, but is normal for extreme athletes. "Rather than get nervous as we got faster, I get calmer," she explained. "When it's life or death, all the static goes away, everything slows down. I can't explain it. It's a magic that happens.

"Maybe it's my ADD. Maybe it's the hypnotherapy, visualization, and neurofeedback I did. And of course, maybe it's also Maximum Overload. It gave me absolute confidence that I had the extra power to push harder and longer than I ever had before. And absolute confidence that we will break the record next year."

Klesges believes that the USRDA of 1,200 milligrams of calcium is too low for athletes exercising over an hour each day, and that supplementation is a must. Getting enough calcium through diet would be difficult. Most sports drinks have little to no calcium. A basketball player practicing hard for 2 hours would have to drink 33 pints of Gatorade's Endurance (12 milligrams of calcium per 16 ounces) a day. The riders in Nichols' study would have to drink 200 pints a week—or consume 12 to 15 cups of yogurt or milk.

Even if they did, keep in mind that cyclists don't cue bone growth like weight-bearing basketball players. So they absolutely need to lift weights and run or jump rope to get the skeletal overload and impact—as did Holland. Along with his cycling, the bike builder takes 1,200 mg of daily calcium supplements and does three 4-mile runs and weight sessions a week. It's paying off, as his bone density has risen 1 to 2 percent each year since his first DXA scan for Nichols' study. Unfortunately, he believes he's an anomaly, seeing few of his cohorts change their eating or exercise habits despite widespread awareness of the issue.

"It's out of sight, out of mind," he says. "They can't see their bones thinning and can't project into the future, so they don't worry. Not me."

IN CONCLUSION

You need muscle—and the only way to get it is lifting weights. If you hate the gym, get over it; there's no other option. Cyclists are lucky, in a way; they not only can derive huge benefits from weight training, but now have a have a highly-motivating, anecdotally-proven, sport-specific plan to follow. Maximum Overload gives weight training a purpose, promising to improve your health, your fitness, and your cycling—in the long run and the short run.

In the long run, Maximum Overload will reverse the muscle-wasting effects of aging that starts in your 30s and accelerates every decade. It'll stop the dangerous bone-density deterioration and early-onset osteoporosis that is caused by aging and a single-sport focus on cycling. It'll help avoid the effects of hormone-wrecking aerobic monotraining. It'll fix your cycling-corrupted posture, improve your balance, melt weight off your belly, prevent injuries, and assure uninterrupted training by strengthening the muscles around the joints to provide cushioning and alignment. When you're old, it'll stop you from falling and breaking your hip. At any age, pretty, robust muscles burn a lot of calories and help you lose weight. They serve as immune-supporting metabolic reservoirs that aid your recovery from traumatic accidents and major surgeries better than your withered peers. Maximum Overload will even allow you to ride less, reducing the chance of burnout, boredom, and traffic injuries. It's safe to say that Maximum Overload can keep you riding years longer, even decades longer.

And if you really want to go faster in the next 60 or 90 days, push your Maximum Sustainable Power (MSP) through the roof, stay superstrong on the last climb of the day, wow your riding buddies, and maybe even get on the podium, it'll do that, too.

ENDNOTES

CHAPTER 6

1   R. J. Godfrey, Z. Madgwick, and G. P. Whyte, "The Exercise-Induced Growth Hormone Response in Athletes," *Sports Medicine*, vol. 33, no. 8 (February 2003): 599–613.

2   Martin J. Gibala et al, "Short-Term Sprint Interval versus Traditional Endurance Training: Similar Initial Adaptations in Human Skeletal Muscle and Exercise Performance," *Journal of Physiology*, vol. 375 (September 2006): 901–11.

3   Amy M. Taylor-Mason, "High-Resistance Interval Training Improves 40-km Time-Trial Performance in Competitive Cyclists," *SportScience*, vol. 9 (2005): 27–31. http://www.sportsci.org /jour/05/amt-m.htm

4   Tudor O. Bompa, *Periodization Training for Sports*, 2nd edition (Champaign, IL: Human Kinetics, 2005).

5   Jonathan Esteve-Lanao, Carl Foster, Stephen Seiler, and Alejandro Lucia, "Impact of Training Intensity Distribution on Performance in Endurance Athletes," *Journal of Strength and Conditioning Research*, vol. 21, no. 3 (August 2007): 943–49.

6   Roy M. Wallack, "Beware the Black Hole," *Outside*, December 3, 2010. https://www .outsideonline.com/1853156/beware-black-hole

CHAPTER 7

1   "The Big Fat Surprise: Why Butter, Meat and Cheese Belong in a Healthy Diet (& What They Don't Tell You About The Mediterranean Diet)," BenGreenfieldFitness.com podcast interview, Feb 2017, https://bengreenfieldfitness.com/2017/02/the-big-fat-surprise-why-butter-meat-and -cheese-belong-in-a-healthy-diet/.

2   Dariush Mozaffarian,MD, DrPH and David S. Ludwig, MD, PhD, "Lifting the Ban on Total Dietary Fat,"*JAMA* 313, no. 24 (2015): 2421-22. doi:10.1001/jama.2015.5941.

CHAPTER 8

1   O. Vikmoen et al, "Strength Training Improves Cycling Performance, Fractional Utilization of VO_2 Max and Cycling Economy in Female Cyclists," *Scandinavian Journal of Medicine and Science in Sports*, vol. 26, no. 4 (April 2016): 384–96.

2   K. Beattie et al, "The Effect of Strength Training on Performance in Endurance Athletes," *Sports Medicine*, vol. 44, no. 6 (June 2014): 845–65.

3   B. R. Ronnestad and I. Mijika, "Optimizing Strength Training for Running and Cycling Endurance Performance: A Review," *Scandinavian Journal of Medicine and Science in Sports*, vol. 24, no. 4 (August 2014): 603–12.

4   J. Louis et al, "Strength Training Improves Cycling Efficiency in Master Endurance Athletes," *European Journal of Applied Physiology*, vol. 112, no. 2 (February 2012): 631–40.

5   P. Aagaard et al, "Effects of Resistance Training on Endurance Capacity and Muscle Fiber Composition in Young Top-Level Cyclists," *Scandinavian Journal of Medicine and Science in Sports*, vol. 21, no. 6 (December 2011): e298–307.

6   A. Sunde et al, "Maximal Strength Training Improves Cycling Economy in Competitive Cyclists," *Journal of Strength and Conditioning Research*, vol. 24, no. 8 (August 2010): 2157–65.

7   Linda M. Yamamoto et al, "The Effects of Resistance Training on Road Cycling Performance among Highly Trained Cyclists: A Systematic Review," *Journal of Strength and Conditioning Research*, vol. 24, no. 2 (February 2010): 560–66.

8   L. L. Ploutz et al, "Effect of Resistance Training on Muscle Use During Exercise," *Journal of Applied Physiology*, vol. 76, no. 4 (April 1994): 1675–81.

9   J. F. Nichols, J. E. Palmer, and S. S. Levy, "Low Bone Mineral Density in Highly Trained Male Master Cyclists," *Osteoporosis International,* vol. 14, no. 8 (August 2003): 644–49.

10   Roy M. Wallack, "Why You Need to Bone Up," *Bicycling,* vol. 45, no. 2 (March 2004): 50–56. http://secondsummertours.com/Articles/stronger-than-ever.pdf

11   F. U. Niethard and A. Gussbacher, "Rapid Boss Loss in High-Performance Male Athletes," *Sports Medicine Digest,* vol. 18, no. 20 (1996).

12   F. Campion et al, "Bone Status in Professional Cyclists," *International Journal of Sports Medicine,* vol. 31, no. 7 (July 2010): 511–15.

13   D. W. Barry and W. M. Kohrt, "BMD Decreases over the Course of a Year in Competitive Male Cyclists," *Journal of Bone and Mineral Research,* vol. 23, no. 4 (April 2008): 484–91.

14   J. F. Nichols and M. J. Rauh, "Longitudinal Changes in Bone Mineral Density in Male Master Cyclists and Nonathletes," *Journal of Strength and Conditioning Research,* vol. 25, no. 3 (March 2011): 727–34.

15   S. E. Warner, J. M. Shaw, and G. P. Dalsky, "Bone Mineral Density of Competitive Male Mountain and Road Cyclists," *Bone,* vol. 30, no. 1 (January 2002): 281–86.

16   Robert C. Klesges et al, "Changes in Bone Mineral Content in Male Athletes," *Journal of the American Medical Association,* vol. 276, no. 3 (July 1996): 226–30.

ACKNOWLEDGMENTS

We have many people to thank for helping us get this book to the finish line.

FROM JACQUES:

I want to thank everyone whose influence throughout my life has made me a better coach. It is amazing how all these lessons greatly impact what you are capable of accomplishing.

My Father and Mother, who never quit and taught me to do the same and together gifted me with a wonderful childhood.

My high school wrestling coach *Roger Renfro.* He gave me a great example of what makes a great coach, and I use those lessons daily. It showed me how much impact a coach can have on an athlete's life, both in the short term and the long term.

Mark Sisson for all his support and guidance. His generous contributions on an ongoing basis the introduction to DZ as well as his friendship and insight.

I am grateful for the crucible of sport. Without it my life would be so different. Win or lose it is within the elegance of struggle where beauty lies and lessons are learned.

FROM ROY:

Jacques DeVore, the first guy I'd ever met to build a logical, organized plan for weight training (which I'd always done myself and promoted as a quality-of-life activity) that is specifically designed to make cyclists go faster (which is the only way to get them to do it).

Bill Strickland, *Bicycling* Editor-in-Chief, who instantly "got" the premise of Maximum Overload when I emailed him the proposal, labeled it a "game changer," and ultimately green-lighted the project to Rodale's book-publishing arm.

Rodale Books executive editor **Mark Weinstein**, for his straight talk and support throughout the project.

My son **Joey,** who encouraged me to shrug-off early rejections and milder offers from other publishers, refocus and rewrite my pitch, and aim for the perfect fit and deal, which happened.

Paleo-movement leader **Mark Sisson,** who introduced me to Jacques and and forced me to learn about diet, which probably plays an even bigger role than exercise in achieving disease-free good health and longevity.

Phil Campbell, author of *Ready, Set, Go! Synergy Fitness*, whose succinct, practical and brutally effective Sprint 8 workouts and research taught me a lot about interval training's endurance, weight-loss and hormone benefits and is referenced in many of my articles and books.

Andy Petranek, my *Fire Your Gym* coauthor, friend and CrossFit guru, who dispensed some key strength-training knowledge that helped me write about this program's unique exercise regimen.

The late, great **Bill Katovsky**, *Triathlete* magazine founder, serial entrepreneur, creative juggernaut, and all-round hilarious guy who got me back into writing books in 2004 when he called one day and said, "You know those stories you're always telling me about running into Hollywood celebrities on your bike? I have an agent. Let's write a book called *Bicycle Sex.*" That became the first edition of *Bike for Life.* I'm truly bummed I won't hear his opinion on this one.

The "Black Hole" guys—**Stephen Seiler, PhD** and **Carl Foster, PhD**—elite sports-science academic researchers whose landmark studies on the importance of recovery to performance and health is *the* key to effective training for everyone. Their "Go Hard, Go Easy" construct has been the basis of several of my articles and book chapters, including Chapter 6 here.

Dr. Jeanne Nichols, San Diego State University professor whose 2003 landmark study on the disturbing osteoporosis-cycling connection led me to write probably my most important story ("Why You Need to Bone-Up," *Bicycling* 2004) and super-charged my life-long interest in athletic longevity.

John Howard, the legendary three-time Olympic cyclist, Ironman winner, world speed record holder and super-coach, the very first person I interviewed as a rookie cycling writer in 1987, who took the challenge I presented to him over the phone in late 2015 and ultimately gave us huge proof that this program worked in the person of the 147.7-mph woman, Denise Mueller.

Finally, thanks to **Denise Mueller**, not only for setting the first woman's land speed record in September 2016, putting cycling back in the news in a good way and giving me a lot to write about, but for keeping me fit. Using the email reports she regularly would send of all her Maximum Overload workouts, I competed against her twice a week and finished this book in the best shape of my life.

ABOUT THE AUTHORS

Jacques DeVore is the founder of the Sirens & Titans Training Centers in West Los Angeles and Santa Barbara, a Certified Strength and Conditioning Specialist, and licensed as an expert USA Cycling Coach. DeVore is the creator of the Maximum Overload training plan. A former collegiate wrestler, DeVore has successfully trained cyclists and triathletes with this program, including pro-rider Dave Zabriskie. He lives in Los Angeles and Santa Barbara, California.

Roy M. Wallack is a health-and-fitness columnist for the *Los Angeles Times*, former editor of *Triathlete, Bicycle Guide,* and *California Bicyclists* magazines, and long-time contributor to *Outside, Bicycling, Runner's World, Competitor, Westways, Consumer's Digest,* and other publications. He's written eight books, including *Bike for Life: How to Ride to 100, Run for Life, The Traveling Cyclist,* and *Barefoot Running Step-by-Step.* A former collegiate wrestler, Wallack has traveled the globe by bike and competed in some of the world's toughest endurance challenges, including the Eco-Challenge, Paris-Brest-Paris, the Badwater Ultramarathon, and his true love, multi-day mountain bike stage races, including the TransAlp Challenge, BC Bike Race, and Costa Rica's legendary La Ruta de los Conquistadores. An inductee in the 24 Hours of Adrenalin Hall of Fame, he lives with his family next to the bike path in Irvine, California.

INDEX

Boldface page references indicate illustrations. <u>Underscored</u> references indicate tables or boxed text.

Explosive Walking Lunge, 46, 47–48,
86, **87**
Reverse Lunge with Overhead Press,
111, **111**
Suitcase Carry/Farmer's Walk, 108, **108**
in upper-body strength test, 115
Waiter's Walk, 109, **109**
Dynamic warm-up, 56–64
about, 57–58
check-in using, 57
Cowboy Walk, 62, **62**
High-Knee Skip, 64, **64**
Hip Thrust/Glute Bridge, 63, **63**
in the Maximum Overload workout,
138
need for, 51–52, 56–57
sequence for, 57
Sidestep Hip Mobility Lunge with
Arms Up, 60, **60**
Stretch-Band Lateral Side Shuffle, 61,
61
Walking Lunge with Thoracic Spine
Mobility Twist, 59, **59**

E

Eccentric contraction, 20
Endurance
fat as fuel for, 190
improved by weight training, 210, 216
LSD aiding, 174–75, 176
muscle loss with training for, 217
Energy/fuel-burning systems, 165
Exercises. *See* Maximum Overload
exercises
Exercise vs. training, <u>214–15</u>
Explosive Walking Lunge
for Baseline APO Test, <u>40</u>, 129–30
benefits of, 46
instructions for, 86, **87**
psyche-up factor for, 47–48

F

Farmer's Walk, 108, **108**
Fast-twitch muscle fibers, 209, 210
Fat, body, 192, 198
Fat, dietary. *See also* Primal or paleo diet
benefits of eating, 198–99, 204–5
body fat not caused by, 198

as clean burning, 176, <u>179</u>, 180, 193,
196–97
Dr. Oz's reversal on, 204–5
as endurance fuel, 190
Framingham Heart Study and, 203–4
fueling activities with, 189
government position on, 8, 200,
202–3, 206
processed oils, 190, 191
rise and fall of the low-fat diet, 202–5
teaching your body to use as fuel,
196–97
weight loss aided by, 192–93
Fat-burning
diet's affect on, 189–90, 195
explanation of, <u>178–79</u>
increased by LSD, 175, 176, <u>179</u>
by slow-twitch muscle fibers, <u>178</u>
stopped by carbs and oils, 191
testosterone boosted by, 219
Foam Roller T-Spine Overhead Reach,
119, **119**
Foam Roll the Hip Flexors, 125, **125**
Form, improving, xi, 19–20
Framingham Heart Study, 203–4
Frequency for routines
intervals, 172
Maximum Overload workout, 136, 152
off-season training, 150

G

Gap, the, xv, 12–13
Glutes, exercises engaging
Bulgarian Split Squat, 84, **84**
Classic Box Jump with a Step-Down,
93, **93**
Classic Kneeling Hip Flexor Stretch,
124, **124**
"Deep" Push Press/Thruster, 88, **89**
Explosive Walking Lunge, 86, **87**
Hex/Trap Bar Deadlift and Dumbbell
Deadlift, 76, **77**
High-Knee Skip, 64, **64**
Hip Thrust/Glute Bridge, 63, **63**
Reaching Lunge, 82, **83**
Reverse Hypers, 66, **66**
Romanian Deadlift, 78, **79**
Single-Leg Crossover Plyo Bench
Jump, 92, **92**

power output on normal riding vs., 168–70

quality vs. quantity for, 167

workout time reduced by, 166

J

Jordan, Michael, 10

Jumps

  APO jump test, 115–16, **116**

  Classic Box Jump with a Step-Down, 93, **93**

  Single-Leg Crossover Plyo Bench Jump, 92, **92**

  Standing Broad Jump, 116, **116**

K

Knee mobility, 126

Knee stability exercises

  Bulgarian Split Squat, 84, **84**

  One-Leg Stand, 110, **110**

Kyphosis

  described, 98–99

  in Howard, 99–101, **100**

  Lat Pulldown counteracting, 72, **72**

L

Land speed records, xix, 2, 224, 227–29

Lateral stabilizers, Cowboy Walk working, 62, **62**

Lat Pulldown, 72, **72**

LeMond, Greg, 8

Long slow distance (LSD)

  challenge of, 185

  for easy workouts, 174, 175

  endurance aided by, 174–75, 176

  fat-burning increased by, 176, 179

  importance of getting it right, 175, 176–77

Low-carb diet. *See* Primal or paleo diet

Lower back, exercises engaging

  Hex/Trap Bar Deadlift and Dumbbell Deadlift, 76, **77**

  Reverse Hypers, 66, **66**

  Romanian Deadlift, 78, **79**

  Tabletop, 107, **107**

Lower-body power exercises, 85–93

  about, 85

Classic Box Jump with a Step-Down, 93, **93**

"Deep" Push Press/Thruster, 88, **89**

Explosive Walking Lunge, 46, 47–48, 86, **87**

reps and sets for, 137–38

rules for, 136–37

Single-Leg Crossover Plyo Bench Jump, 92, **92**

strength exercises aiding, 74

strength vs. power and, 85

Wall Ball, 90, **91**

Lower-body strength exercises, 74–84

  about, 74–75

  Bulgarian Split Squat, 84, **84**

  choosing which to do, 74

  finding starter weights for, 133

  Hex/Trap Bar Deadlift and Dumbbell Deadlift, 75, 76, **77**

  in the Maximum Overload workout, 139–40

  power exercises aided by, 74

  power vs. strength and, 85

  Reaching Lunge, 82, **83**

  reps and sets for, 134

  risk with, 74

  Romanian Deadlift, 78, **79**

  rules for, 133–34

  Single-Leg Press, 80–81, **81**

  Suitcase Carry/Farmer's Walk, 108, **108**

  weight for, 134

Lower-body strength test, 114

Low-fat diet, 202–5

LSD. *See* long slow distance

Lunges

  deadlifts vs. walking lunges, 32–34, 37–38

  Explosive Walking Lunge, 46, 47–48, 86, **87**

  favorites for cycling-specific power, 74

  improved by deadlifts, 39

  in lower-body strength test, 114

  Reaching Lunge, 82, **83**

  Reverse Lunge with Overhead Press, 111, **111**

  Sidestep Hip Mobility Lunge with Arms Up, 60, **60**

  Walking Lunge with Thoracic Spine Mobility Twist, 59, **59**

M

N

Natural diet. *See* Primal or paleo diet

O

Off-season training
  calendars, 154–55, 156–57, 160–61
  frequency for, 150
  goals, 153–54, 157, 159
  replacing cycling workouts, xvii
  starting Maximum Overload, 150
  week at a glance, 153
  Weeks 1 to 4, 153–56
  Weeks 5 to 8, 157–58
  Weeks 9 to 12, 159–60
Oils, processed, 190, 191
Olson, Timothy, 194
O'Neill, Shaquille, 15–16
One-Leg Stand, 110, **110**
Osteoporosis, 208, 219–22, 223. *See also*
    Bone health
Overhead Ball Chop, 113, **113**
Overhead Band Pulses, 120, **120**
Overload. *See also* Weight training
  defined, xiv, 4, 18–19
  eccentric and concentric contraction
    in, 20
  heavy vs. light weights for, 168–69
  increased by resting between mini-
    sets, 26–27
  raising in Phase 2, 144–45
  Roman calf raise, 19
  supercompensation with, 19
Overload protocol, xvii
Oz, Mehmet, 204–5

P

Paleo diet. *See* Primal or paleo diet
Palms, heat controlled through, 25
PAP, 173
Pelvic-Tilt Plank, 67, **67**
Performance
  core temperature's effect on, 25
  equalizing leg strength for, 80
  heavy vs. light weights and, 168–69,
    209–10, 211
  impact of all muscles on, 65
  improved by better recovery, 181

improved by paleo diet, 198
improved by using fat as fuel, 191
improved by weight training, 17, 18,
    209, 210–11
intervals for improving, 167
power-to-weight ratio and, 187
reduced by Black Hole training, 180
second-half deterioration, 5–6, 29
supercompensation and, 19
Phase 1—Weeks 1 to 4
  goals of, 152
  Maximum Overload workout, 132–34
  MSP workout, 142–43
  off-season training, 153–56
Phase 2—Weeks 5 to 8
  goal of, 152
  Maximum Overload workout, 134–35
  MSP workout, 144–45
  off-season training, 157–58
Phase 3—Weeks 9 to 12
  goal of, 152
  Maximum Overload workout, 135
  MSP workout, 145, 148
  off-season training, 159–60
Physio Ball Reverse Hypers
  basic instructions, 66, **66**
  in core strength test, 115
Planks
  Plank, 106, **106**
  Static Plank and Pelvic-Tilt Plank, 67, **67**
Postactivation Potentiation (PAP), 173
Posture
  kyphosis, 98–101, **100**
  Lat Pulldown correcting, 72, **72**
  mobility drills aiding, 54
  T-spine corrective exercises, 121–22
Power. *See also* Absolute Power Output
    (APO)
  cycling sweet spot and, 35–37
  deadlifts vs. walking lunges for, 37–38
  formula for, 35, 128–29
  improved by Maximum Overload, xi,
    224
  improved by weight training, 209, 210
  lower-body power exercises, 85–93
  maintaining as the goal of training, 29
  as missing link for cyclists, 3
  output on intervals vs. normal riding,
    168–70
  ratio of weight to, 187, 215
  reduced by overheating, 26

Weight training. *See also* Maximum
Overload exercises
aerobic training aided by, 4
antiaging effect from, 213–15, 216
benefits for cyclists, xii–xiii, 17–23
bone health improved by, 21, 208,
222–23, 230
cyclists' resistance to, xii, xv, 9, 12–13,
15, 49–50
eccentric and concentric contraction
in, 20
evolution in sports, 8–11
exercise vs. training, 214–15
fast results with, xi, 18
gains from simple additions, 209
heavy vs. light weights for, 168–69,
209–10, 211
hormones boosted by, 23, 165, 218–19
overload achieved by, xiv
performance improved by, 17, 18, 19,
209, 210–11
power improved by, 209
prevalence throughout sports, 9, 14,
15–16
quality of life improved by, 208
replacing a road workout with, 213
research on, 209–12

retirement postponed by, 10
road training enhanced by, 20–21
Russian advances in, 16–17
speed improved by, 18, 208–9
supercompensation and, 19
three-sets-of-6-to-8 orthodoxy, 24
Zabriskie's improvement from, ix–x
Wheat, 202
Williams, Brad, 146–47
Workouts. *See* Maximum Overload
workout; Maximum Sustainable
Power (MSP) workout
Workout time
for Maximum Overload workout, 128
reduced by intervals, 166
reduced by weight training, 22–23, 213
reduced with Maximum Overload, xi

Z

Zabriskie, Dave
condition before starting, xviii
crash and retirement of, 193–94
diet's affect on, 188–89
performance improvements by, ix, x,
xiv, 30
weight lifting by, ix–x